The Consumer's Guide to Health Care

The Consumer's Guide to Health Care

Francis V. Chisari, M.D.
Robert M. Nakamura, M.D.
Lorena Thorup, B. S., R. N.

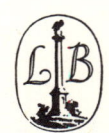

Little, Brown and Company—Boston–Toronto

COPYRIGHT © 1976 BY FRANCIS CHISARI AND ROBERT NAKAMURA
"WHAT YOU NEED TO KNOW BEFORE CHOOSING A NURSING HOME"
COPYRIGHT © 1976 BY LORENA THORUP

ALL RIGHTS RESERVED. NO PART OF THIS BOOK MAY BE REPRODUCED IN ANY FORM OR BY ANY ELECTRONIC OR MECHANICAL MEANS INCLUDING INFORMATION STORAGE AND RETRIEVAL SYSTEMS WITHOUT PERMISSION IN WRITING FROM THE PUBLISHER, EXCEPT BY A REVIEWER WHO MAY QUOTE BRIEF PASSAGES IN A REVIEW.

FIRST EDITION
T 05/76

LIBRARY OF CONGRESS CATALOGING IN PUBLICATION DATA

Chisari, Francis V
  Consumer's guide to health care.

  Includes bibliographical references.
  1. Medical care. 2. Physician and patient. 3. Medicine—Specialties and specialists. 4. Voluntary health agencies—United States. 5. Consumer education. I. Nakamura, Robert M., joint author. II. Title. [DNLM: 1. Consumer participation. 2. Delivery of health care—U.S. WB50 AA1 C45]
RA410.5.C44   362.1   75-38950
ISBN 0-316-13908-4

Designed by Susan Windheim

Published simultaneously in Canada
by Little, Brown & Company (Canada) Limited

PRINTED IN THE UNITED STATES OF AMERICA

Preface

OVER THE YEARS we have spent many evenings answering questions raised by our friends and relatives about the adequacy of their health care. We continue to be appalled by how uninformed and naive the average American is concerning the best way to utilize the services of the medical profession and the health care industry for the maintenance of his health. Compounding this problem is a lack of communication partially created by the timidity of the patient to question the judgment of his physician.

Despite the current trend of consumerism which has encouraged institutional reform, quality control and increased availability of medical services, the individual patient remains poorly equipped to influence the quality of his health care. With this in mind we have written this book in an attempt to give the consumer-patient the insight necessary to deal effectively and personally with his health care providers.

The authors wish to thank Ms. Lorena Thorup, B.S., R.N., for contributing the chapter on nursing homes which represents an expansion of a pocket pamphlet written by Ms. Thorup for the San Diego Chapter of the American Association of University Women.

This book would not have been possible without the tireless and excellent secretarial assistance of Mrs. Cleo-Mae Mrozek. We thank Mr. Berkeley Rice for his editorial advice, wit and consumer's perspective. The credit for conceiving this book belongs to our relatives and friends whose questions prompted us to outline its chapters. The momentum to proceed and complete the book, however, was provided by the enthusiasm, encouragement and assistance of our wives.

Introduction

Problems Facing the Consumer in the Health Care Field

HAVE YOU EVER —
- moved to a strange city or suburb and had to select a physician or clinic solely on the word-of-mouth recommendations of new neighbors?
- wondered what kind of doctor you should see for a given problem?
- wished you could review a physician's credentials before you make an appointment?
- wanted to know where you could find reliable and understandable information about your illness?
- questioned the quality of your medical care?
- worried about the adequacy of your health insurance program and what provisions you should make for the not uncommon catastrophic illnesses which can drain your resources?
- wondered what recourse you have for grievances

against your physician or hospital, or what constitutes a valid grievance?

These questions represent just a sampling of the problems and dilemmas facing the American consumer in the health care field today.

As in the purchase of any other valuable commodity, the consumer has a vital interest in the quality of the product and the price he pays for it. In the health care field, however, the "commodity" is virtually invaluable and the consumer's interest in making the purchase is self-evident. In commercial terms this creates a seller's market in which a prudent individual should exercise caution. The consumer-patient must entrust the care of his health, his most vital possession, to a major industry and a technology much too complex to fully comprehend. He must deal with this industry and technology through trained professional representatives who, in crass terms, depend on the occurrence of his misfortune for their livelihoods. There is hardly a situation imaginable in which the consumer is potentially at such a tremendous disadvantage.

And yet, despite these formidable odds, the American consumer has within his reach health care of a very high quality. In the vast majority of instances his health care providers serve him well. Nevertheless, the consumer-patient is often ignorant of the services available to him and unable to evaluate the quality of the care he receives. This book will provide the reader with the tools he needs to solve these problems.

Contents

INTRODUCTION
  Problems Facing the Consumer in the Health
  Care Field ... vii

1. **THE QUALITY OF YOUR MEDICAL CARE:
   YOU CAN IMPROVE IT** ... 3
     What should you know about your illness? ... 4
     What should you know about your physician? ... 7
       Competence ... 9
       Availability and coverage ... 14
       *Hospital affiliations and teaching
       appointments* ... 15
       Office policies ... 17
       Physician's personality ... 18

CONTENTS

2. WHAT ARE YOUR RIGHTS AS A PATIENT? — 20
   The patient's Bill of Rights — 21

3. WHAT YOU SHOULD KNOW BEFORE CHOOSING A PHYSICIAN — 32
   Characteristics of the inadequate and/or unconcerned physician — 36
   Group versus solo practice — 39
   What about the osteopath? — 41

4. THE SPECIALIST AND WHAT HE CAN DO — 43
   (Under each Board listed below the requirements for certification and special skills of the specialist are described.)
   The American Board of Allergy and Immunology — 45
   The American Board of Anesthesiology — 47
   The American Board of Colon and Rectal Surgery — 48
   The American Board of Dermatology — 49
   The American Board of Family Practice — 50
   The American Board of Internal Medicine — 51
   The American Board of Neurological Surgery — 59
   The American Board of Nuclear Medicine — 60

The American Board of Obstetrics and Gynecology	61
The American Board of Ophthalmology	62
The American Board of Orthopedic Surgery	63
The American Board of Otolaryngology	64
The American Board of Pathology	65
The American Board of Pediatrics	66
The American Board of Physical Medicine and Rehabilitation	69
The American Board of Plastic Surgery	70
The American Board of Preventive Medicine	71
The American Board of Psychiatry and Neurology	73
The American Board of Radiology	76
The American Board of Surgery	78
The American Board of Thoracic Surgery	79
The American Board of Urology	81
5. WHAT YOU SHOULD KNOW ABOUT YOUR LOCAL HOSPITAL	82
What types of hospital are available in your community?	82
Function	83
Ownership	85

xii CONTENTS

      What are the essential features of a modern acute care hospital?   89

6. EMERGENCY MEDICAL CARE   97
      What constitutes a true emergency?   97
      What should you do in the wake of an emergency?   99
      How should you get to the emergency room?   103
      What to expect when you arrive at the emergency room   104
      Standard operating procedure in the emergency room   107
      How to prepare for emergencies before they occur   108

7. MEDICAL SERVICES AVAILABLE FROM COMMUNITY HEALTH AGENCIES   111
      (General information and specific services available to patients are discussed under each organization.)
      Local health services   112
          Visiting nurse association   112
          Home health aides   113
          Meals-on-Wheels   114
          Department of public health   115

CONTENTS xiii

Medical supply rental services	115
Health and medical information by telephone	116
Consumer medical education on television	116
National Voluntary Health Associations	116
Overall structure and general purpose	118
Support	118
Objectives	119
Organization	119
National Council on Alcoholism, Inc.	120
Allergy Foundation of America	121
The Arthritis Foundation	121
The National Foundation — March of Dimes	122
The National Society for the Prevention of Blindness, Inc.	123
Fight for Sight, Inc.	124
The National Association for Visually Handicapped	125
The American Foundation for the Blind	126
The American Cancer Society	127
Leukemia Society of America, Inc.	129
The United Cerebral Palsy Associations, Inc.	130
The National Cystic Fibrosis Research Foundation	131

xiv CONTENTS

The American Diabetes Association, Inc.	132
The Epilepsy Foundation of America	133
The National Easter Seal Society for Crippled Children and Adults	134
The American Heart Association, Inc.	135
The National Hemophilia Foundation	136
The National Council for Homemaker — Home Health Aide Services, Inc.	138
The National Kidney Foundation, Inc.	138
Planned Parenthood — World Population	140
National Multiple Sclerosis Society	141
The Muscular Dystrophy Associations of America, Inc.	142
The Myasthenia Gravis Foundation, Inc.	143
The National Paraplegia Foundation	144

8. WHAT YOU NEED TO KNOW BEFORE CHOOSING A NURSING HOME 146
   Before you look 149
   Ready to look: what to look for. 151
   The building 151
   Personnel 154
   What you need to know about personnel 155
   Care of patients 158

Facilities in rooms	163
Sanitation	164
Safety	165
Recreation	167
Food	168
Costs of a nursing home	170
What you can do to help the nursing home and the patient	172

9. THE CONSUMER AND THE COST OF PRESERVING HIS HEALTH ... 174
   Generic versus brand name drugs: cost versus quality ... 174
   Anticipating the cost of your medical care ... 180
   Essentials of an adequate health insurance plan ... 183

10. ADVICE TO THE DISSATISFIED CONSUMER ... 185

APPENDIX: ... 191
   Home Medical Library ... 193
   Pocket Health Record ... 197

The Consumer's Guide to Health Care

1

The Quality of Your Medical Care: You Can Improve It

DESPITE MANY EXCESSES and distortions, American "consumerism" has focused attention on the consumer's right to know as much as possible about the product or service he pays for. This pertains to health care just as to breakfast cereals. The consumer has the right to expect the provider of medical services to demonstrate his credentials of training and experience, his availability when needed, his awareness of current developments and his fee on an hourly or some other reasonable basis.

Implicit in this philosophy is the consumer's responsibility to learn about the validity of professional standards, the requirements for licensure and certification, and the ability of certifying agencies to ensure that current and ethical practices are being employed. He must know enough to be able to understand the significance of the information he has at hand. Unfortunately, the consumer often does not know how to evaluate the quality of medical services. For example, the "cure" is perhaps the most easily identified parameter of medical excellence. Yet many common diseases run their course unaffected by any form of therapy, good or bad. Thus, "cure" is not synonymous with quality nor does lack of "cure" imply inadequate care. Furthermore, although a physician's bedside manner and aura of self-confidence can put a patient at ease, these qualities alone do not assure good care. But most consumers restrict their evaluation of health care quality to these factors because they do not know how else to go about it. The major objective of this book is to attempt to correct this situation. Indeed, this is essential to enlightened consumerism. Without it the consumer must accept on faith the information available to him. When one must evaluate the quality of the health care he receives the stakes are much too high to rely on faith alone.

WHAT SHOULD YOU KNOW ABOUT YOUR ILLNESS?

This question is one of the major problems facing the health care consumer. If he knew with certainty the nature of the illness for which he sought medical attention, and its appropriate therapy, he would have no difficulty evaluating the quality of the care he received. However, even the simplest and commonest illnesses can masquerade as the exotic and vice versa, and many complex factors must be considered in order to reach a decision about the appropriate form of therapy. Since the average layman has neither the time nor the inclination to acquire the knowledge necessary to evaluate each illness as it arises he must rely on the judgment of a trained medical professional.

This does not imply, however, that he must passively accept the diagnosis and treatment without question. After all, no one has more interest in the accuracy and wisdom of those decisions, nor more at stake than the patient himself. It therefore makes good common sense for the patient to ask his doctor a number of critical questions about his illness. These include:

1. The certainty of the diagnosis.
2. The usual course of the illness and what impact it may have on his activity.
3. The reasons for the choice of the specific form of therapy and the side effects of any prescribed medication.

If satisfactory answers are not forthcoming the patient should purchase one of the several good home health guides, a textbook of clinical pharmacology and a medical dictionary and review for himself the specific diagnosis rendered by his physician, and the particular medication (if any) prescribed. He can also contact one of the many voluntary health agencies discussed in Chapter 7 which publish reliable information about a large variety of diseases. If he has any further questions he should not hesitate to consult again with his physician.

In most instances this process may not be necessary but it will always be desirable for a number of reasons. First of all, the patient's independent reading will probably confirm his doctor's opinion and reaffirm the patient's confidence in his physician. Second, it will help to educate the patient about his illness and the importance of following his doctor's advice. Third, it should make the patient aware of side effects of drugs which his physician may have neglected to tell him about. So many drugs are available today, each with a great number of adverse effects, that few physicians can be aware of all of them, even though by law and by the tenets of good medical practice they should. Finally, on occasion the physician's opinion will be wrong. Certainly this should come as no surprise to anyone who recognizes that all physicians are fallible human beings and that the art and science of medicine is still in its infancy, with vast areas of collective professional ignorance. The physician depends a great deal on the information provided by the patient to reach a diagnosis, to correct problems as they arise, and to evaluate the efficacy of therapy. The patient can therefore improve the accuracy of this process if he is adequately informed about his illness and medication.

We recognize that many patients would rather leave all decisions about their health care to the physician of their choice. Indeed, many patients are unwilling or unable to assume the responsibility of participation in this particular decision-making process. Furthermore, many patients need to have absolute trust and faith in their chosen physician for their own peace of mind. We don't deny the merits of this attitude. We are sure, however, that when all else is equal the informed patient is more likely to receive better quality care than the uninformed.

We also anticipate that some physicians may view our suggestions with skepticism. Some will say that a little knowledge is dangerous. Others will predict an increasing number of "nuisance calls" if patients adopt these practices. Still others will propose that these suggestions may erode the public's confidence in the medical profession. Our reply to all these observations is a forceful "Yes . . . but they will foster physician-patient communication and patient education both of which are essential and frequently neglected ingredients in quality patient care."

WHAT SHOULD YOU KNOW ABOUT YOUR PHYSICIAN?

It is a harsh fact of life that we can do little to preserve our health other than to provide ourselves with adequate nutrition, shelter and clothing, and to avoid the known hazardous and noxious elements of our environment. Susceptibility to most human disease is usually beyond our control. We can, however, generally exert full and absolute control over the choice of the physician into whose care we entrust the preservation and maintenance of our good health. If for no other reason, therefore, this choice should be made on as solid a basis as possible and only after a thorough and systematic evaluation.

Nevertheless, most people wait until some illness. frequently unexpected and sometimes quite grave, forces them into a doctor's office before they do anything to assure themselves of his competence. If for some reason they then find him not quite up to their expectations, it is all too easy for them to lament the deficiencies of the medical profession in general and to condemn the human failings of the physician in particular. Certainly the medical profession faces many serious problems and very few physicians have the intellect of a Nobel Prize winner or the compassion of Saint Luke. But in large measure the consumer himself must accept responsibility for his dissatisfaction. If he had made the effort to investigate the physicians in his community at a leisurely and careful pace when he enjoyed the luxury of good health, he would have a vastly greater chance of being satisfied with his medical care when he most needed it.

Unfortunately many people haven't analyzed the elements of quality health care well enough to be able to know what to look for in a physician. They frequently don't know where to get the information they may want to know or they are too timid to come right out and ask a physician or his staff the questions they may have on their minds.

We suggest that you begin this search and analysis on a first-priority basis when you move into a new community, or today, if you presently are dissatisfied with your physician or if you don't have one. We must emphasize at the outset that there is nothing mysterious or difficult about this. It will take some time and will require at least one visit to a physician's office. In no way will this process guarantee you everlasting health. We are confident, however, that the consumer who follows this advice will be better able to assure himself of the quality of the services he obtains.

COMPETENCE

In the evaluation of any tradesman or professional, this critical and essential element is usually the most difficult to determine without knowledge of the field or experience with the person. However, a physician must reach a number of milestones and fulfill certain fairly rigid professional requirements before he is acknowledged by his colleagues to have reached any one of several levels of competence in his field. Since this information is public knowledge the consumer can learn much about his prospective physician, sometimes even before he calls a doctor's office.

1. Is the Physician Licensed to Practice Medicine in Your State?

This is not at all as ridiculous as it appears. In a recent survey conducted in a major metropolitan area, fully 15 percent of the medical practitioners listed in the telephone directory were not licensed to practice medicine. A phone call to your State Board of Medical Examiners is all that is necessary to find out this essential fact.

2. How Much Formal Postgraduate Medical Training Has He Received?

Upon graduation from medical school most states require for licensure a minimum of one year of postgraduate training in a hospital approved by the Joint Commission on Accreditation of Hospitals as well as successful performance in examinations administered either by the National Board of Medical Examiners or the particular State Board. Once these requirements have been met a physician can enter practice. Many physicians elect to spend usually two or more additional years in what is called residency training, learning, in greater depth, the intricacies of a particular specialty such as Family Practice, Internal Medicine, Pediatrics, and so forth. Some physicians go even further and may spend one or more years after residency in what is called fellowship training in an even more specialized discipline such as Cardiology, Infectious Diseases, or Gastroenterology.

When a physician successfully completes the training requirements in one of these areas he becomes eligible to take an examination in that field administered by the appropriate specialty board. He is then called "board eligible." If he passes the exam he is judged to be proficient in that area and is awarded a certificate which attests to the fact that he is "board certified." Many physicians post these certificates in their offices along with diplomas, licenses and the like for your review, and they should serve not to impress you but to inform you of their level of formal training. If no certificates attesting to training beyond internship are displayed it means either that the physician, for any number of reasons, had no further training — if he did he failed to fulfill the strict requirements for board certification — or he chooses not to display them. In any event if you don't see them you owe it to yourself to ask him to review for you his postgraduate training, which is one of the few objective criteria by which you can judge your doctor's fund of knowledge. You don't even have to visit a physician's office, however, to obtain this information. It is available from the State or County Medical Society, the AMA *Physicians Reference Listings* and the *Directory of Medical Specialists*, copies of which should be available in your public library.

We do not mean to imply that a physician who has not pursued a formal postgraduate training program need be any less competent in his area than a qualified specialist is in his. Indeed, many super-specialized physicians may be unfamiliar with the proper management of even common illnesses in fields other than their own and would, therefore, be wisely avoided if you are in need of a generalist. On the other hand, many physicians with little or no training beyond internship are highly capable individuals who have managed to keep abreast of modern medical developments and are well suited to the management of the majority of illnesses. But make no mistake about it, the licensing and certification procedures are not infallible. In some respects inadequate and unqualified physicians manage to slip by at all levels. The likelihood, however, decreases with increasing length of training if for no other reason than the fact that such individuals are monitored by more than one faculty and for a longer period of time. So if all else is equal, when you are looking for a physician, you are likely to select one with greater knowledgeability if you choose one with more formal training. Likewise, in view of the ever-increasing complexity of medical science, the specialist is indispensable when diagnoses are obscure, management of an illness requires delicate juggling of body chemistry, and therapy is new and dangerous.

3. Is He Making an Effort to Remain up to Date in His Knowledge of Medical Theory and Practice?

This information can only be obtained from the physician himself or his staff and you should not be too timid or embarrassed to ask. Medicine is developing so rapidly that if a physician stands still for one year he falls back two. The questions to ask are "What medical journals do you read?" and "How often do you attend medical lectures and seminars?" The physician's professional reading should not be confined to magazines devoted to the economics and politics of medicine. He should be reading at least one general technical journal (like the *New England Journal of Medicine*, *Archives of Surgery*, etc.) and, if he claims to be proficient in a specific area, at least one specialty journal (such as the *American Journal of Cardiology*). Furthermore, he should be attending lectures and seminars devoted to subjects appropriate to his practice on a frequent basis. These are offered by local hospitals and universities, and often sponsored by the AMA, various specialty boards, and county and state medical societies. They are invaluable methods of refreshing one's memory of things learned but forgotten, and of catching up with new developments. There are, however, numerous "conferences" in exotic, faraway places which are little more than thinly disguised vacations. So ask him what he reads and what his last conference was about. If he dodges the question or becomes cool or irate you've probably hit a sore spot and may be dealing with an outdated physician no matter what his age.

4. What about Experience, Analytical Ability and the Capacity to Discriminate between the Important and the Irrelevant Aspects of a Case?

These are very difficult questions and there is probably no good objective method to form an accurate opinion short of observing the physician over a period of years. Certainly, and obviously, these are traits which are usually acquired as one grows older, but in no way does increasing age guarantee nor does youth preclude the existence of these traits. Collectively they could be called wisdom, and we know of no foolproof, quick and easy way to detect it. Perhaps a reasonably accurate assessment of these factors can be obtained from the doctor's other patients. Directed and specific questions relating to frequency of complications, length of hospitalization, number of laboratory tests, frequency of office visits, frequency of referral to other doctors and so on are often useful probes to elicit this important information.

AVAILABILITY AND COVERAGE

No matter how intelligent, well-trained, compassionate and wise a physician is, he is of little use to you unless he or someone he designates is available when necessary. It therefore is critical to ask him or one of his staff:

1. How often and how willing is he to see or speak with you when you need him?
2. Does he make house calls and if not, why not?
3. Is he willing to give telephone consultations?
4. Is there a time during the day that he specifically sets aside for phone calls?

This practice allows the patient to call for advice without fear of interrupting the doctor and assures the physician of fewer interruptions during the rest of the day.

5. Does he make it a point to personally meet his patients at the local emergency room and treat them himself or does he delegate that responsibility to an emergency room doctor . . . or nurse?
6. How often and for how long does he visit hospitalized patients?
7. Who covers for him when he is not on call at night or

when he is on vacation and what are that doctor's qualifications?
8. How often is he off duty?
9. How long will you have to wait for a "routine" and for an "urgent" office visit?

This information can be easily given by the physician's nurse or receptionist over the phone or in person. Insist on it because the need for a physician doesn't end with office hours.

HOSPITAL AFFILIATIONS AND TEACHING APPOINTMENTS

The hospital or hospitals with which a physician is affiliated play a vital role in the quality of the care you receive. It is likely that a competent physician will be affiliated with a hospital that provides him with the facilities he requires to render superior medical care. Such facilities are not always available, however, especially in inner city and rural areas where many highly reputable physicians choose to live and work. Although even the most sophisticated medical centers cannot make provisions for every conceivable emergency and complication, even the most rudimentary hospital facility should have the capacity to handle all common emergencies efficiently.

Ask your prospective physician about the adequacy of the hospital pharmacy, whether there is an emergency cart equipped for the management of cardiac and respiratory arrest, if there is at least a portable cardiac monitoring apparatus and someone present on each nursing shift who is trained in its use. Ask him about the experience of the surgical staff and the anesthesiologist and what kind of surgery can be performed there. Does he have confidence in the accuracy of the reports he receives from the pathologists and radiologists or does he send his patients elsewhere for lab work? If you know you have a specific ailment like emphysema ask him whether the hospital is equipped with the necessary ventilatory assist devices and a respiratory care technician in case you get into serious trouble and need immediate and intensive care. Is there an intensive care unit and trained staff to operate it? Ask him how long the waiting list is for admission to the hospital, whether there is a physician present in or near the hospital at all times and how quickly he could get you to a different hospital if you were critically ill and could not receive adequate care at the first hospital.

Finally, ask him if he is also affiliated with any medical school as a visiting physician with responsibility for teaching medical students, interns and residents. There is no better way for a physician to remain current and aware of new developments or to refresh his memory of the basic physiology of disease than to be constantly peppered with questions from younger colleagues. Indeed, one of the great services these young physicians make to the consumer-patient is to keep his personal physician aware of how much he has forgotten.

OFFICE POLICIES

These are the ground rules the physician sets for the smooth and orderly functioning of his practice. Most of these questions can be answered by the office nurse or receptionist and frequently are found on printed cards or brochures in the waiting room.

The following information should be available to you:

1. What are his office hours?
2. Are new patients accepted?
3. Which evenings and weekends is he on call?
4. How can he be reached in an emergency?
5. Does he see children, make house calls, or charge for telephone consultation?
6. What is the cost of an initial visit, a routine physical, a follow-up visit, minor surgical procedures, and laboratory procedures such as chest x-ray, EKG, urinalysis, blood count, and throat culture?
7. Is prepayment a condition before a patient is seen?
8. Does he participate in Medicare, Medicaid, Blue Cross or other third party payment programs?
9. How large is the practice?
10. Is more than one patient scheduled every fifteen minutes?
11. Is the patient charged for broken appointments?
12. If the doctor is occupied with an emergency does the waiting room just fill up or are patients given new appointments?
13. Is there adequate clerical help to assist in filling out insurance forms?

The answers to these questions will give you a reasonably good idea about how pleasant your relationship with the physician and his office will be.

PHYSICIAN'S PERSONALITY

This brings us to the last important question you should try to answer before choosing a physician. When you have checked his background, spoken with him and his staff, and perhaps even had a screening physical exam, do you like him? Although certainly this is not an essential element in terms of the quality of the care you will receive, it is nonetheless important. At the very least you should be convinced of his intellectual honesty, his ability to communicate his observations and recommendations, and his capacity to instill confidence in his decisions. Without these qualities even the most brilliant physician can't be a healer because his patient is not likely to follow his advice.

In summary, we have recommended the following in this chapter: The consumer must actively evaluate his physician before he selects him and throughout the course of the doctor-patient relationship if he is to have any impact on the quality of the health care he receives. Prior to selecting a physician the consumer can determine for himself the educational background and availability of the physician, the nature of his office and hospital facilities, the ground rules of the physician's practice and some basic aspects of his personality. This should be done as soon as the consumer moves to a community or becomes dissatisfied with his current physician. It is ideally done while he is healthy and not pressured by circumstances to find one in a hurry. It will take the investment of time, energy and the price of an initial office visit. If the consumer is still not satisfied, he may have to repeat the process until he is. The investment will be well made, however, for it is actually a form of insurance policy on his most precious and irreplaceable asset: his health. He should also play an active role in educating himself about each illness as it arises so that he will be better able to communicate with his physician and understand the rationale behind the prescribed therapy. Yes, the consumer can influence the quality of the health care he receives, but he must be willing to do a little to get a lot in return.

2

What Are Your Rights As a Patient?

WHEN YOU ESTABLISH a professional relationship with a physician you acquire a number of important rights as a patient. You must know what these rights are and be ready to exercise them if you intend to affect the quality of the medical care you receive.

In 1972 the American Hospital Association adopted a set of resolutions which has come to be called the patient's "Bill of Rights." Although this is not a legal document it does clearly define the rights and privileges which you, the patient, should demand from your health care provider.

Let us take these principles, one by one, and discuss the impact they can have on your medical care.

WHAT ARE YOUR RIGHTS AS A PATIENT?

The Patient's Bill of Rights

1. "The patient has a right to considerate and respectful care."

For the most part the meaning of this statement is self-evident. Certainly a patient's sex, race, religion or socioeconomic status should not affect the manner in which he is treated. Nonetheless, all of these factors, and many others, influence each patient's personality, his response to his illness, and his expectations from the medical establishment. In return, the individual health care provider will respond to each patient as an individual molded by these factors.

In this setting, personality clashes will unavoidably occur and may adversely affect the quality of the patient-physician relationship. When this happens you should discuss it openly with your doctor and try to work out a solution. Occasionally the solution will be to transfer your care to another, more compatible, physician. This usually can be done with little difficulty or embarrassment.

2a. "The patient has the right to obtain from his physician complete current information concerning his diagnosis, treament and prognosis in terms the patient can be reasonably expected to understand. When it is not medically advisable to give such information to the patient, the information should be made available to an appropriate person on his behalf."

It goes without saying that the patient or his family must be kept informed of the current status of his health, especially in the presence of longstanding, progressive illness. Furthermore, the implications of any significant change in fitness for work, suitability for vigorous recreation, or longevity, must be made known to enable the patient or his family to plan for the future. Much needless anxiety can be prevented by asking your physician for a periodic assessment of your condition. It is your right to have this information provided in terms you can understand. Physicians spend much of their time talking and writing in medical jargon and sometimes it is difficult for them to express themselves in simple terms. Don't be afraid, therefore, to ask the doctor to explain his findings more clearly if you don't understand what he has said.

2b. ". . . He has the right to know, by name, the physician responsible for his care."

This is especially important if you are hospitalized in an institution which is heavily staffed by residents and interns. These young physicians-in-training usually spend no more than three or four months working in any one area of the hospital. Although they usually are supervised by one or more fully trained physicians, even the latter may rotate from one service to another.

Under these circumstances you should find out if one particular physician will be assigned to your case for an extended period of time. Although this is very desirable, it frequently isn't possible, especially in some large, urban, municipal hospitals. You may therefore be assigned to the care of a particular outpatient clinic where you may see a different doctor each time you visit. In this type of situation the only thread of continuity is your medical record in which each doctor records his findings and lists his recommendations. This is a less than desirable situation not only because of the way it fragments your medical care but also because the records can be lost and are sometimes illegible.

It is one of the great ironies and tragedies of the American medical system that these conditions usually affect the economically deprived patient from the inner city who is hospitalized in a university-affiliated teaching hospital where the most advanced and modern medical facilities are available. In contrast, the well-to-do patient from the suburbs usually can afford to have his own personal physician, but frequently lives too far from a university hospital to derive any direct or immediate benefits from its existence.

3. "The patient has the right to receive from his physician information necessary to give informed consent prior to the start of any procedure and/or treatment. Except in emergencies, such information for informed consent should include but not necessarily be limited to the specific procedure and/or treatment, the medically significant risks involved, and the probable duration of incapacitation. Where medically significant alternatives for care or treat-

ment exist, or when the patient requests information concerning medical alternatives, the patient has the right to such information. The patient also has the right to know the name of the person responsible for the procedures and/or treatment."

We emphasize here that an explanation of a procedure and the risks involved is not enough. The implications of *not* doing the procedure should also be discussed, as should alternative procedures which might be substituted. We recognize that giving an explanation that is complete but at the same time totally understandable to a patient is not an easy task. Such an explanation cannot be only verbal. It must be complete with appropriate diagrams and pictures and ample opportunity should be given for the patient to ask questions. The risks of the procedure or treatment should be thoroughly discussed. Some physicians fear that by talking about risks they will discourage the patients from undergoing treatment that they, the physicians, feel is necessary. Nonetheless, although the doctor should provide information and opinions, it is the patient who must consent.

Recently, an organization of physicians interested in health communication problems published a set of books called *DOCUBOOKS*™ for patient use. Each of these books describes a specific treatment or procedure (such as breast surgery), including its benefits and risks as well as alternatives. These books are meant to supplement the physician-patient discussion. Each contains a document which the patient is encouraged to sign when he has read and understood the information. Hopefully these books will help the patient to participate more actively in making the decisions which affect his health care, thereby lessening the misunderstandings which sometimes lead to malpractice suits. There are currently more than twenty-five titles available. Information about these books may be obtained from:

> HEALTH COMMUNICATIONS, INC.
> 52 W. Kellogg Boulevard
> St. Paul, MN   55102

4. "The patient has the right to refuse treatment to the extent permitted by law and to be informed of the medical consequences of his action."

You may, at any time, refuse treatment for any particular ailment. This is true regardless of your reasons, e.g., loss of confidence in your physician, religious beliefs and the like. Some patients terminally ill with an incurable illness refuse treatment which would prolong their lives because it would also prolong their suffering and add to the financial burdens on their families.

There are two important restrictions on this right, however, which vary somewhat from state to state. In general terms they are stated as follows. First, if you are declared mentally incompetent by a panel of physicians and judged to be so by the courts, a physician may treat you against your will on the assumption that you would allow treatment if you were mentally sound. Second, you may not refuse treatment for your child if he is a minor, on religious grounds. The legal assumption here is that you are making a religious, not a medical, decision for the minor and that he is entitled to modern medical care until he is legally responsible for his own decisions.

5. "The patient has the right to every consideration of his privacy concerning his own medical care program. Case discussion, consultation, examination and treatment are confidential and should be conducted discreetly. Those not directly involved in his care must have the permission of the patient to be present."

This includes everyone from insurance carriers to physicians or nurses who are not providers of his care.

6. "The patient has the right to expect that all communications and records pertaining to his care should be treated as confidential."

There are certain public health regulations which require communicable disease information to be reported. Other institutions or individuals, such as schools, potential employers, insurance companies, must have the written permission of the patient in order to receive copies or summaries of his records. The patient, on the other hand, is entitled to thorough access to his medical records. This means that when you change physicians, for whatever reasons, all of your medical records can and should be transferred to that physician promptly at your request. This can save you the expense, inconvenience and risk of having to repeat many diagnostic procedures and provides the new physician with a thorough history of your health status.

7. "The patient has the right to expect that within its capacity a hospital must make reasonable response to the request of a patient for services. The hospital must provide evaluation, service, and/or referral as indicated by the urgency of the case. When medically permissible, a patient may be transferred to another facility only after he has received complete information and explanation concerning the need for and alternatives to such a transfer. The institution to which the patient is to be transferred must first have accepted the patient for transfer."

The patient can be reasonably assured of these rights if he is hospitalized in an accredited hospital (see Chapter 5) which has a variety of board certified specialists (see Chapter 4) on its staff. In small communities with only a few doctors and modest hospital facilities the range of services available will be restricted. Because of this the patient in such a situation should expect to be referred elsewhere for the management of difficult problems. This in no way should detract from the esteem in which he holds his local physician or clinic. Indeed, the wise physician knows when his expertise and the facilities available to him are insufficient to provide the best possible care for his patients.

8. "The patient has the right to obtain information as to any relationship of his hospital to other health care and educational institutions insofar as his care is concerned. The patient has the right to obtain information as to the existence of any professional relationships among individuals, by name, who are treating him."

Basically this means that the patient is entitled to know whether his hospital is affiliated with one or more of a variety of medical institutions which can materially affect the quality and thoroughness of his care. These institutions include medical schools, research foundations, specialized treatment centers, extended care facilities and so on.

Furthermore, the patient should know whether the physicians who are contributing to his care in a hospital are in business together (group practice) or individually (solo practice). Although group practice offers many advantages to both the patient and the physician, it can limit the number of consultants from which the doctor may choose for his difficult cases. For example, let us say you are seeing a general internist because of a heart problem and he decides you should be evaluated by a cardiologist. If the general internist is a member of a group which includes a cardiologist in its membership you probably will be referred to that cardiologist even if he is not the most qualified one in the area.

We mention this only for your information so you will be able to judge the services you receive for yourself. Indeed, we endorse fully the concept of group practice. We only mean to point out that it is not without its limitations.

9. "The patient has the right to be advised if the hospital proposes to engage in or perform human experimentation affecting his care or treatment. The patient has the right to refuse to participate in such research projects."

The Department of Health, Education and Welfare has issued a document for the protection of human subjects which discusses human experimentation as it affects the patient's care. Any experimentation must be approved by the hospital's committee on human research and requires approval of each patient studied.

The patient has every right to refuse to participate in such research projects. Before he agrees to participation in any research project he should be informed of the

a) purposes of the study
b) benefits, if any, which he may derive from joining the study
c) departures from ordinary practice entailed in the study
d) risks, dangers and inconveniences to which he may be exposed
e) right to drop out of the study at any time.

The patient should definitely understand the alternatives to participation in the experiment.

10. "The patient has the right to expect reasonable continuity of care. He has the right to know in advance what appointment times and physicians are available and where. The patient has the right to expect that the hospital will provide a mechanism whereby he is informed by his physician or a delegate of the physician of the patient's continuing health care requirements following discharge."

All this means is that the patient is entitled to continuing care. Once a physician has accepted a patient into his practice it is the doctor's responsibility to follow the patient's condition as often and as long as necessary for the patient's well-being.

On occasion a physician may decide that he no longer wishes to provide care to a particular patient. This is one of his rights as a physician. He must, however, notify the patient far enough in advance so that a new doctor can be found and the patient's records can be transferred.

11. "The patient has the right to examine and receive an explanation of his bill, regardless of the source of payment."

In fact, many physicians now post their fees for various and specific services (such as "brief office visit," "complete physical examination"). We feel that this is ideal since it allows the patient some choice, on still another level (i.e., a financial one), regarding his plan for health care. The patient, furthermore, has the right to receive an *itemized* list of charges from both a physician and a hospital, even if an insurance company will be paying the bill.

12. "The patient has the right to know what hospital rules and regulations apply to his conduct as a patient."

This includes everything from policies regarding visitors to whether he will be allowed to smoke. A hospital's regulations regarding patient conduct are generally printed in pamphlet form and are presented to the patient on admission.

In summary, you have a great deal at stake when you trust the maintenance of your health to the care of a physician. In return for this trust you acquire a number of very important rights. You must exercise these rights if you intend to do more for yourself than sit on the sidelines while your physician tries to defend you from the onslaught of disease. You must not be afraid to assert these rights when necessary nor should you be intimidated by the apparent wisdom and learning of your doctor. Most important of all, you should insist that you be educated about your illness and the measures necessary to treat it. Armed with this information you will have no difficulty assuring yourself that your remaining rights will be honored. Without this knowledge you are a passive bystander and you will never really know whether your rights have been violated. The choice is yours.

3

What You Should Know Before Choosing a Physician

IN ORDER TO DERIVE any benefits from the health care system it is obviously necessary to first gain entry into the system. The logical and most efficient method is to establish a professional relationship with a physician who can direct you through the maze of available services. The importance of selecting that physician wisely cannot be overemphasized.

Many persons are unable to decide what kind of doctor is best suited to their particular needs. Some patients prefer to select a different specialist for each specific medical problem that may arise. Others prefer to place the total responsibility for every aspect of their health care into the hands of a single physician. Although each of these alternatives is attractive and has some merit, neither arrangement is suitable for the delivery of comprehensive medical care.

The ever-increasing complexity of the biomedical sciences makes it impossible for any single physician to provide the best possible care for all of his patients' ailments. For the same reasons, no layman can adequately select the specialist most suited to his particular needs by himself. We believe that optimal medical care can be obtained only from a team of health care providers, each with his own special area of competence. Such a team must have a leader, a manager so to speak, who selects the appropriate "players" at the proper time, who coordinates and directs their efforts and guarantees that the best interests of the patient are served at all times.

In other words, we suggest that you place the responsibility for the comprehensive management of your health care into the hands of a generalist. You and he together should decide whether you need the services of a specialist and who should be selected among the ones available.

When we use the term "generalist" we mean one of three types of physicians: the general (or family) practitioner, the internist, and the pediatrician. By "specialist" we mean any one of a wide variety of physicians who have obtained additional training in a relatively narrow area and who, therefore, are likely to be able to provide you with specific services not ordinarily available from the generalist. It should be apparent that both types of physicians are essential for thorough and comprehensive medical care and that neither one alone can serve you optimally without the other. Let us see an example to illustrate this point.

Mr. X is a sixty-year old banker who is in relatively good health although his blood pressure is higher than it should be. He has recently noticed a feeling of tightness in his chest when he walks uphill on cold windy days.

High blood pressure is a common condition which affects many different organs and requires the regular attention of a physician, who will try to minimize or prevent these effects by a program of weight reduction, diet and drugs. Such services can be provided by most competent internists and general practitioners. When a potentially serious complication like chest pain arises, the following questions will arise as the generalist considers the patient's situation:

1. What is the cause of the chest pain; is it due to heart disease, bronchitis or something else?
2. If heart disease is responsible, is it due to atherosclerosis (hardening of the arteries), aortic stenosis (a narrowing of one of the heart's valves), a combination of these or something else?
3. If it is due to atherosclerosis, are there abnormalities of the blood lipids (fats like cholesterol and triglycerides) which can be controlled by diet and drugs?

Up to this point many generalists are perfectly capable of handling the situation. From the information they obtain by taking a careful history and performing a thorough physical examination and relatively simple laboratory tests, they can pinpoint the problem and begin appropriate treatment. Other generalists, however, are uncomfortable with such problems and feel that their patients are better served if they send them straight to a specialist in heart disease (cardiologist) as soon as they think the patient's symptoms are cardiac in origin. There is one further question, however, which every generalist must ask which normally results in referral to a specialist:

4. Is the problem surgically correctable?

Some heart conditions are potentially reversible with appropriate surgical treatment. In order to determine if this is so the blood vessels, valves and inner chambers of the heart must be examined by cardiac catheterization. This procedure is beyond the scope of the generalist and is usually performed by a cardiologist. Depending on the findings the cardiologist, in consultation with the generalist and the cardiac surgeon, decides whether the patient's heart disease can be treated surgically.

Such a team approach is essential for the proper management of many problems as common as high blood pressure and heart disease. It should be apparent that the generalist and specialist each have something important to contribute to the patient's care. It should be equally apparent that the patient can greatly influence the quality of his medical care depending on how wisely he selects his generalist.

As we stated earlier, general medical care is usually provided by the family practitioner, the internist and the pediatrician. Since the availability of these physicians will vary from community to community you may or may not have an assortment of generalists to choose from. The only physician in some communities may be a lone general practitioner. Other communities may be fortunate enough to have several general practitioners as well as a variety of internists and pediatricians. If you live in one of these latter communities you may have trouble deciding which type of generalist to choose. (In Chapter 4 we outline the particular qualifications of each of these physicians to help you with this decision.) Once the type of generalist has been chosen, you may then have to decide which one of the several who practice in your area to select.

We have already discussed those qualities which characterize the competent physician. Now let us consider the other side of the coin: namely, how to recognize the inadequate physician regardless of his field. Hopefully, once you know what to seek and what to avoid in a physician, these choices will be made more easily and more wisely.

CHARACTERISTICS OF THE INADEQUATE AND/OR UNCONCERNED PHYSICIAN

1. He doesn't spend enough time with you.

It takes time for the doctor to determine what the possible causes of your chief complaint are, to ask all the questions necessary to narrow the range of diagnostic possibilities, to perform the appropriate physical examination, to formulate a final or tentative diagnosis, to explain to you what his conclusions are and to answer any questions you might have. Therefore, the first visit for even a relatively minor complaint should last at least fifteen minutes, and often must be considerably longer depending on the nature of the patient's symptoms. Follow-up visits to check on progress can be thorough, however, even if they are relatively brief.

2. He takes an inadequate medical history.

Your doctor *must* listen and record your serious complaints before any medical evaluation can begin. He must then ask a number of questions to help give him a clear idea of the nature of your illness and the medical setting in which it occurs. This verbal exchange is the doctor's *most important and powerful diagnostic tool*. A few peremptory questions are certainly no substitute for a careful, methodical and thorough medical history which includes the following general areas:

a) *Chief complaint*. The reason the patient has chosen to visit the doctor. Usually recorded in the patient's own words.
b) *History of the present illness*. Information regarding the duration of the symptom, factors which aggravate and alleviate or are associated with it, and similar questions are typical of this section of the medical history.

c) *Review of systems.* The status of each body organ is reviewed by a long series of questions designed to detect malfunction that might have been ignored, forgotten or unnoticed by the patient.
d) *Past medical history.* Past illnesses, operations, vaccinations, medications, injuries and infections are reviewed.
e) *Family history.* Hereditary predisposition to certain diseases is considered in this section.
f) *Personal and social history.* Habits such as tobacco, alcohol and drug ingestion, and the patient's occupation and life-style are reviewed.

All of these areas should be covered in a general way during one of your first visits to a doctor so he can have a health profile with which to compare any subsequent changes. During later visits for other complaints you should be asked selected questions, pertinent to your complaints, from most of these categories. If you aren't questioned in this manner it is rarely because the nature of your illness is self-evident; rather it is usually because the doctor is in a hurry.

3. He performs an inadequate physical examination.

There are very few disorders that affect one part of the body without also affecting other adjacent or related structures. For this reason it is imperative that a reasonably comprehensive examination be performed in order to properly evaluate any isolated complaint. Beware, therefore, of the doctor who rushes through the physical examination or only examines one part of your anatomy. Obviously, this is not the case when the complaint is a head cold in a season full of head colds, or a sprained wrist or stubbed toe; but many medical problems are more complex than that. Too simple an examination may well indicate that the doctor is not being thorough and you, the consumer, are being cheated of the medical consultation you are paying for.

The remaining qualities are self-explanatory.

4. He doesn't adequately explain his reasons for performing special tests or the risks associated with them.
5. He doesn't educate you about your illness and explain the importance of adhering to his prescribed treatment.
6. He doesn't warn you about the common and serious side effects of the medicine he prescribes for you.
7. He doesn't arrange for necessary follow-up to check the efficacy of his treatment.
8. He doesn't answer your questions to your satisfaction.
9. He rarely refers his patients to another doctor for consultation and is offended when you ask for a second opinion.
10. He doesn't have hospitalization privileges at one or more local hospitals.

Group Versus Solo Practice

At this point it is appropriate to consider the advantages of group versus solo practice from the patient's point of view. Although the one most important factor which determines the quality of the health care you receive is the competence of your physician, we believe that the doctor in group practice is better equipped to provide superior care than an equally competent solo practitioner.

As a member of a group, the physician has ready access to formal and informal professional consultation which can save the patient a considerable amount of time and inconvenience. Because of the variety of physicians in the group the patient may obtain a wider range of medical services under one roof and he usually is guaranteed around the clock medical coverage by physicians who have immediate access to his records. The records themselves can be maintained in a more systematic form than by the solo practitioner simply because most of the consultations and tests are performed by members of the group who use the same records. Perhaps the most important aspect of group practice as far as the patient is concerned is the fact that his doctor's methods are constantly observed and scrutinized by the other physicians in the group. This peer pressure is a vital and potent stimulus which usually encourages the physician to remain up-to-date and employ only accepted medical principles.

The superior physician can manage his patients quite well without the additional support provided by the group. If all other considerations are equal, however, you stand a better chance of receiving higher quality medical care from a physician in group practice than from the same physician in practice alone.

What About the Osteopath?

There are practitioners other than physicians who are legally and professionally permitted to use the title "doctor." Among these groups the consumer is most likely to encounter the osteopath, the podiatrist and the chiropractor. Since this book addresses itself to those practitioners who are qualified and licensed to provide *complete* medical care we will restrict our discussion to doctors of osteopathy.

Dr. Andrew T. Still founded the first school of osteopathy in 1892 after the loss of three of his children during an epidemic of meningitis. Dissatisfied with the limited services which conventional medicine could offer to the patient, Dr. Still formulated the theory that many diseases were caused by musculoskeletal imbalance. He postulated that the improper alignment of bones, especially in the spinal column, produces nervous system malfunction and circulatory disturbances which ultimately result in a wide variety of disease states. He therefore advocated the manipulation and alignment of bones and joints as the primary form of treatment.

Given the rudimentary state of orthodox medicine at that time, it is easy to understand the frustration that led Dr. Still to develop his theories and the enthusiasm with which they were received by his patients. However, with the advent of major advances in the biomedical sciences the osteopathic view of disease has changed considerably. In fact, at the present time the courses taught in schools of osteopathy and schools of medicine are virtually identical, although considerable emphasis on the structural basis of disease still exists.

Because of these similarities in training, and since the requirements for admission to schools of osteopathy and schools of medicine are so similar, osteopaths are now eligible to pursue postgraduate education in training programs accredited by the American Medical Association. Many osteopaths and the American Osteopathic Association (AOA), however, prefer to retain the separate identity of the practice of osteopathic medicine. For this reason, among others, many osteopaths train and practice exclusively in AOA-sponsored hospitals.

The doctor of osteopathy (D.O.) is qualified to practice medicine and surgery on an equal footing with doctors of medicine (M.D.). The consumer should therefore evaluate the D.O. with the same criteria he would use to judge an M.D. You will find over 75 percent of osteopathic physicians in general practice and many of them are excellent family physicians. Be sure to find out, however, whether your potential D.O. restricts himself to the consultative services of only osteopathic specialists and hospitals, which may not be able to provide you with the full range of medical services because of their relative scarcity.

4

The Specialist and What He Can Do

MOST OF WHAT IS KNOWN today about the human body, its normal functions, and the mechanisms which produce disease, has been learned in the past fifty years. Furthermore, the rate at which new facts have been uncovered has accelerated with each decade. Currently, there are over one hundred scientific journals devoted to the publication of new medical discoveries. So many manuscripts are submitted to these journals for publication that it usually takes between six and twelve months before an article actually appears in print. No physician has the time or the ability to keep abreast of all these developments.

Consequently, many physicians choose to confine their practices to a single area of human disease — a specialty. This enables them to remain abreast of current information in that specific field. It stands to reason, however, that if a physician restricts his practice to only one aspect of medicine he will be less well informed about other medical specialties. He will thus tend to refer patients who have medical problems outside his field of interest to other specialists. This results in highly competent but fragmented medical care and creates the need for the well-trained generalist to "bring it all together" for the patient.

The patient should be warned, however, that a physician need not have advanced training in a particular medical specialty in order to call himself a "specialist." All he need do is restrict his practice to that particular area. For example, a doctor can list himself in the Yellow Pages of your telephone directory as a specialist in a given area of medicine without having had the training necessary to be officially recognized as a specialist in that field (see discussion of postgraduate training and board certification in Chapter 1). This physician is less likely than a certified specialist to have the fund of knowledge necessary to solve a particular problem in that area.

The consumer-patient should therefore have some understanding of what safeguards the medical profession provides for him in the form of officially recognized specialties and formal examining boards in various medical specialties. As listed in the 1974 edition of the *Directory of Medical Specialists*, a publication of the American Board of Medical Specialties, there are currently twenty-two well-defined areas of medical practice which are closely scrutinized by twenty-two specialty boards. Each board is composed of specialists qualified in the particular field represented by that board and is approved by the

Council on Medical Education of the American Medical Association. The purpose of each board is, first, to determine if physicians who voluntarily apply for certification have been adequately educated in the particular field; second, to administer comprehensive examinations to determine the competence of each applicant, and third, to certify that those physicians who have fulfilled these requirements are indeed competent. The successful applicant is awarded a certificate attesting to his achievement and he is listed in the *Directory of Medical Specialists*. The patient, therefore, can determine for himself whether his physician is an officially recognized specialist simply by checking the *Directory*, which should be found in the public library.

During his years of postgraduate training the specialist acquires unique skills and additional knowledge which make him a particularly valuable and essential member of the practicing medical community. In the section that follows we shall list the twenty-two officially recognized Medical Specialty Boards, summarize their requirements for certification as listed in the *Directory of Medical Specialists* and discuss the particular talents which their members can bring to bear on specific medical problems.

THE AMERICAN BOARD OF ALLERGY AND IMMUNOLOGY

REQUIREMENTS FOR CERTIFICATION
1. Certification as a specialist by the American Board of

Internal Medicine, the American Board of Pediatrics (see below) or certification in Internal Medicine or Pediatrics by the Royal College of Physicians and Surgeons of Canada.
2. Plus at least two years of additional training in Allergy and Immunology.
3. Plus successful completion of the specialty board examination.

NOTE: Requirements 1 and 2 are not necessary if the candidate has had at least ten years of practice principally in Allergy and Immunology under circumstances acceptable to the board.

SPECIAL SKILLS The Allergist-Immunologist is uniquely prepared to deal with such problems as asthma, hay fever, food allergies and a wide variety of other allergic diseases. He can perform and interpret skin tests to determine what is causing the allergy and administer increasing doses ("allergy shots") of the offending agent in an attempt to "desensitize" the patient to that agent and decrease the patient's symptoms. He is specially qualified to evaluate and treat patients who have defective immunological defense mechanisms which make them more susceptible to the development of infections and malignancy. Occasionally these defense mechanisms go awry and attack rather than protect body tissues. This aberration results in the group of "autoimmune" diseases which also can be expertly handled by this specialist. There is a vast area of research called experimental immunology in which the allergist may participate but about which the patient is usually unaware.

THE AMERICAN BOARD OF ANESTHESIOLOGY

REQUIREMENTS FOR CERTIFICATION
1. Applicant must be either a licensed doctor of medicine or osteopathy.
2. Two years of residency in Clinical Anesthesia after which he must pass a written examination.
3. Either one additional year of training or two years of practice at which time he must pass an oral examination.

SPECIAL SKILLS   Most patients think of anesthesiologists only as physicians who "put them to sleep" prior to a surgical operation. In fact, these physicians are vital to the successful outcome of a surgical procedure, since they must be able to support life functions under the stress of anesthesia and surgery. In addition, they are central members of many "cardiac arrest" teams in hospitals, being responsible for the vital respiratory (breathing) function of the critically ill patient. They also are expert in the use of artificial ventilation which is required for the care of patients with severe lung disease. In this capacity they frequently are directors of hospital intensive care units. Furthermore, they can often help the patient with severe and uncontrollable pain by administering local injections to interrupt the transmission of nerve impulses to and from painful areas ("nerve blocks").

THE AMERICAN BOARD OF COLON AND RECTAL SURGERY

REQUIREMENTS FOR CERTIFICATION
1. Applicant must be a licensed doctor of medicine.
2. Four years of training in general surgery.
3. One year of training in colon and rectal surgery.
4. Or, three years of general surgical and two years of colon-rectal surgical training.
5. Or physicians certified by the American Board of Surgery (see below), who limit their practice to colon and rectal surgery and have demonstrated special competence in that field.
6. Successful completion of a written and oral examination in the basic sciences.
7. Successful completion of a practical examination in which the physician is observed in the operating room, on his hospital rounds and in his office.
8. Successful completion of a written and oral examination on the theory and practice of colon and rectal surgery.

SPECIAL SKILLS These physicians are frequently called "proctologists." They are especially qualified to examine and perform surgical operations on the colon, rectum and anus (the lowermost portions of the intestinal tract). The diseases which they commonly encounter are cancer of the colon and rectum, diverticulosis, inflammatory diseases of the colon, colonic and rectal polyps, hemorrhoids, and fissures and fistulas and so on. They are skilled in the use of a tubelike instrument called the proctoscope (or sigmoidoscope) whereby they can directly visualize the inner lining of the rectum where approximately 75 percent of colon-rectal cancer originates. They may also be expert in the use of a new instrument called the colonoscope which is a long flexible tube which, when inserted into the rectum, can be passed with relatively little discomfort through the entire length of the colon. Polyps can be removed through both instruments, thereby avoiding the necessity of surgery in many instances.

THE AMERICAN BOARD OF DERMATOLOGY

REQUIREMENTS FOR CERTIFICATION
1. Applicant must be a licensed doctor of medicine or osteopathy.
2. One year of internship or residency training in another specialty.
3. Three years of residency training in Dermatology.
4. At least six months of additional experience.
5. Successful completion of a written and an oral examination.

SPECIAL SKILLS The dermatologist is an expert in the diagnosis and treatment of disorders of the skin. Although most patients may be familiar with them because of a few relatively common diseases like acne, psoriasis, seborrhea and so on, these physicians are trained to treat a vast array of skin disorders including skin cancer (of many varieties), infections, allergic disorders and so on. Since many diseases of internal organs may manifest themselves as skin disorders long before they are otherwise detectable, the dermatologist is often helpful in the early diagnosis of diseases which originate elsewhere.

THE AMERICAN BOARD OF FAMILY PRACTICE

Currently there are no specific training requirements for certification beyond those required for licensure in a particular state and successful completion of an examination given by the Board.

However, in recent years the Board has encouraged the establishment of residency programs in Family Practice in medical centers throughout the country. These programs usually consist of two or three years of residency during which time the physician gains the experience necessary to diagnose and treat the majority of common illnesses. At the completion of the residency the family practitioner is qualified to handle such diverse problems as the frequently encountered diseases of childhood and adulthood, childbirth, fractures and other injuries and so on.

The family practitioner, therefore, plays an essential role in the American medical community. He is capable of performing a wider variety of services to a more diverse population of patients than any other specialist. Since he can handle most of the problems of all members of a family, he can provide unique insight into many diseases which are inheritable, infectious or stem from emotional conflict within the family unit. He can refer patients who have very complex or obscure diseases to the appropriate specialist but usually can treat these diseases after consultation with that specialist. Perhaps his greatest asset is the fact that he often provides continuing observation of patients who may be afflicted by several chronic diseases. Because of this vantage point he may be able to detect signs of deterioration at an early time when treatment is most likely to be effective.

THE AMERICAN BOARD OF INTERNAL MEDICINE

REQUIREMENTS FOR CERTIFICATION IN GENERAL INTERNAL MEDICINE

1. The applicant must be a licensed doctor of medicine or osteopathy.
2. A minimum of two years of training in general

internal medicine with responsibility for the direct care of patients with diverse medical diseases.
3. A minimum of one additional year of training either similar to the above or in another area related to internal medicine (exceptional instances).
4. Successful completion of a written examination administered by the Board.

REQUIREMENTS FOR CERTIFICATION IN SUBSPECIALTY AREAS
There are a number of special areas (subspecialties) which fall within the scope of general internal medicine. These areas include:

1. Cardiovascular diseases.
2. Endocrinology and metabolism.
3. Gastroenterology.
4. Hematology.
5. Nephrology.
6. Infectious diseases.
7. Medical oncology.
8. Pulmonary diseases.
9. Rheumatology.

REQUIREMENTS FOR CERTIFICATION IN THESE AREAS INCLUDE:
1. Certification in General Internal Medicine.
2. Two additional years of full-time postgraduate education in the subspecialty.
3. Successful completion of an oral or written examination administered by the subspecialty Board.

SPECIAL SKILLS *General Internal Medicine:* The general

internist is trained in the diagnosis and treatment of virtually all the diseases of adults excluding those requiring surgery. In this capacity he is qualified to handle such diverse illnesses as diabetes, high blood pressure, heart disease, emphysema, cancer, a wide variety of infections and many others.

He is not formally trained in the treatment of major injuries but is qualified to handle minor accidents. Like the family practitioner, he is a generalist who is capable and very well suited to the care of a large number of illnesses. He can provide continuing care of patients with chronic diseases. He has been trained in the subtleties of diagnosis; for this reason his surgical colleagues frequently call upon him to help them evaluate patients who have illnesses which might make surgery hazardous or fraught with complications.

The field of internal medicine is very broad and complex. Many internists, therefore, take additional training in specific subspecialty areas to enable them to deal with the especially difficult or exotic problems internists face daily.

Cardiovascular Diseases: This subspecialty deals specifically with illnesses of the heart and blood vessels. The cardiologist has special expertise in the interpretation of the electrocardiogram (EKG) and a working knowledge of various other devices which can monitor heart functions by measurement of sounds and pressure changes produced by the heart on the chest wall and blood vessels. Some cardiologists are also trained in the performance and interpretation of cardiac catheterization.

This is a procedure in which a long, thin tube is inserted into the inside of the heart via a blood vessel in the arm or groin and direct observation of the heart function is possible. These physicians are frequently directors of hospital cardiac care units and are essential members of most open heart surgery teams.

Gastroenterology: The gastroenterologist is an internist who specializes in diseases of the entire intestinal tract, the liver and the pancreas. He is trained in techniques which enable him to directly visualize the upper and lower intestine and to remove tissue from these areas (biopsy) for examination by a pathologist. With an instrument called the panendoscope he can see the lining of the esophagus, the stomach and the duodenum where he may detect evidence of inflammation, stricture, ulcers or tumors. Likewise, with the proctoscope and colonoscope (see section on colon and rectal surgery above) he can examine the lower intestine. With newer instruments he can insert a tube directly into the ducts which connect the liver and pancreas to the intestine to search for stones or cancer. He is also trained in the procedure of liver biopsy in which a needle is inserted, relatively painlessly, through the skin into the liver to remove a small sample of tissue for microscopic examination. Because of his knowledge and technical ability he is an extremely helpful member of the health care team.

Pulmonary Diseases: This specialty is concerned primarily with patients who have lung diseases such as bronchitis, emphysema and cancer. These physicians, like the anesthesiologists, are especially well trained in the use of artificial respiratory machines and in the very complicated aspects of management of the patient with severe lung failure. The pulmonary disease specialist is trained in bronchoscopy. This is a procedure in which a tube is inserted through the mouth into the bronchi, the major breathing tubes, in order to visualize and remove tissue and secretions from the inside of the lung. They are also trained in the use of numerous devices which measure various aspects of lung function in order to detect different forms of lung disease. The pulmonary disease specialist has become increasingly important in this age of atmospheric pollution with its associated effects on our lungs.

Endocrinology and Metabolism: The endocrinologist specializes in diseases of the glands which produce hormones such as insulin, thyroid hormone, adrenalin and the sex hormones. He therefore treats patients with diseases such as diabetes, hyperthyroidism, infertility and so on. He frequently employs sophisticated chemical tests of the blood and urine to measure the level of activity of the endocrine (hormone producing) glands. Because of the vital role these hormones play in virtually every bodily function and because of the delicate chemical balance that must be maintained in patients who have abnormal amounts of hormones, the endocrinologist can be of great assistance in the diagnosis and treatment of these diseases.

Hematology: This specialty is concerned with diagnosis and treatment of patients with diseases of blood and blood-forming organs, especially the bone marrow and spleen. The leukemias and various forms of anemia constitute the bulk of the problems seen by the hematologist. He is trained in methods to obtain samples of bone marrow tissue for microscopic analysis as well as in the interpretation of that tissue. The hematologist is also an expert in diseases which affect the blood clotting mechanism such as hemophilia. He is a student of the specific functions of the various cells in the blood and often plays an essential role in the organization and administration of the hospital blood bank.

Infectious Diseases: The specialist in infectious disease has spent two or more years studying about the incredible number of viruses, bacteria, fungi and parasites which can infect and cause disease in man. He is more knowledgeable than his colleagues about the various manifestations of infection which can mimic almost all human diseases from cancer to stroke. The hospital microbiology laboratory often serves as his base of operations. The infectious disease specialist is trained in the identification of dangerous microscopic organisms and in the use of the powerful drugs available to eliminate them. He is usually the chairman of the hospital infection control committee and often sets the hospital's policy concerning the isolation of patients with contagious diseases, operating room sterile technique and so on. The hospital environment contains more dangerous "bugs" than almost any other location in our society. Since many hospitalized patients are in a weakened state and susceptible to infection, the infectious disease specialist plays a vital role in the care of these patients.

Medical Oncology: The medical oncologist is an internist who specializes in the treatment of patients with cancer. Because of his knowledge of the behavior of the great number of human malignancies he is eminently qualified to evaluate patients who are suspected of having cancer but in whom the diagnosis is not established. Once a particular kind of malignancy is found, the oncologist must determine the extent of the disease, whether and where it has spread, whether it is treatable and he must decide on the best form of treatment. He usually meets frequently with colleagues from the specialties of general surgery and radiotherapy (see below) in order to discuss particular patients and to choose the treatment plan most likely to be effective. He is particularly expert in the choice and administration of the various drugs used in cancer treatment as well as their side effects. He can, therefore, wisely select the drug most appropriate for a particular malignancy and administer it in such a way as to obtain the greatest therapeutic effect with the least possible amount of danger and discomfort to the patient. We therefore recommend that all patients who have cancer satisfy themselves that their physicians have at least consulted with a medical oncologist before treatment is begun.

Nephrology: The nephrologist focuses his attention primarily on the function of the kidneys. He has the knowledge and technical ability to handle the entire spectrum of kidney disease from slight infection to severe uremia. He must understand the way the kidneys excrete and conserve water, minerals, proteins, sugars, drugs and poisons. He is skilled in the procedure whereby a small piece of kidney tissue is removed from the patient using needle biopsy techniques. He can recognize and interpret the abnormal microscopic findings in that tissue. The nephrologist is the director of the Hemodialysis (artificial kidney) unit in the hospital and is responsible for the smooth functioning of that unit. He is also skilled in a process called peritoneal dialysis in which large volumes of fluid are washed into and out of the abdominal cavity via a tube inserted into the abdomen through the skin. Finally, he is an essential member of the kidney transplant team.

Rheumatology: Rheumatology is concerned primarily with diseases which affect the joints such as rheumatoid arthritis, osteoarthritis, gout and so on. The rheumatologist is skilled in the diagnosis of these diseases, which often mimic one another. He can interpret the changes in joint anatomy by physical examination and x-ray techniques. Furthermore, he can withdraw fluid from inflamed joints and analyze it chemically and microscopically. Many of the drugs which are used to treat the various forms of arthritis require careful adjustment of dosage because of potentially dangerous side effects. The rheumatologist is particularly able, because of his training and experience, to regulate the medications so that they are most effective in controlling the arthritis while least likely to produce adverse reactions. He also shares with the immunologist (see Allergy-Immunology, above) an interest in the "autoimmune" diseases mentioned previously.

THE AMERICAN BOARD OF NEUROLOGICAL SURGERY

REQUIREMENTS FOR CERTIFICATION
1. Applicant must be a licensed doctor of medicine.
2. One year of training in general surgery.
3. Four years of training in neurological surgery.
4. Two years of independent practice of neurological surgery.
5. Successful completion of examinations administered by the Board.

SPECIAL SKILLS   The neurosurgeon has a long list of skills each of which is concerned with the diagnosis and treatment of diseases of the nervous system (brain, spinal cord and nerves) and its surrounding bony structures. He can interpret the pattern of electrical impulses generated by the brain by a process called electroencephalography (EEG). He can probe the inner structures of the brain and spinal cord by the injection of radioactive materials (brain scan, etc.), air (pneumoencephalography), and various dyes (myelography). He can examine the structure of the blood vessels in the brain (arteriography) and can evaluate the function of the special sensory organs (eye, ear, touch, etc.) by a number of other techniques. With the aid of all these methods he can frequently determine what a patient's disease is and where it is located in his nervous system. He then can operate to correct or remove whatever is causing the problem. He is trained to perform services such as the removal of a "ruptured disc," the management of serious head injuries, the surgical treatment of severe epilepsy and brain tumors and so on. The many years of training and experience required before he is eligible to take the certifying examination attest to the skill required of him.

THE AMERICAN BOARD OF NUCLEAR MEDICINE

REQUIREMENTS FOR CERTIFICATION
1. The applicant must be a licensed doctor of medicine or osteopathy.
2. Completion of two years of training in either internal medicine, pathology, radiology or another field acceptable to the Board.
3. Two years of residency training in nuclear medicine.
4. Or three to ten years of experience in nuclear medicine plus one to three years of training as above.
5. Successful completion of an examination administered by the Board.

SPECIAL SKILLS The nuclear medicine specialist is uniquely qualified to use radioactive materials (radioisotopes) in the diagnosis and treatment of various diseases. His tools include highly sophisticated equipment which can detect radioactivity in diseased areas of selected organs (liver, thyroid, spleen, lung, brain, bone, etc.) after the injection of small amounts of the radioisotopes into the blood. His knowledge and skills are extremely useful in the treatment of certain diseases of the thyroid gland with radioisotopes. This form of treatment often provides an alternative to the otherwise necessary surgical therapy of these diseases. In addition, the specialist in nuclear medicine frequently serves as the radiation safety officer in a hospital. In this capacity he is responsible for the safe and careful handling of radioactive materials by hospital employees in order to protect hospitalized patients from accidental dangerous overexposure to these agents.

THE AMERICAN BOARD OF OBSTETRICS AND GYNECOLOGY

REQUIREMENTS FOR CERTIFICATION
1. The applicant must be a licensed doctor of medicine.
2. Three years of residency in obstetrics and gynecology.
3. Successful completion of a written examination administered by the Board.
4. At least twelve months of independent practice.
5. Successful completion of an oral examination administered by the Board.

SPECIAL SKILLS The physician trained in obstetrics and gynecology is particularly prepared to deal with problems related to the female genital system. This includes all aspects of childbirth including forceps delivery, cesarean section and abortion. Furthermore, he is a surgeon with the skills necessary to correct or excise diseases of the ovaries, fallopian tubes, uterus and vagina. These include cancer, benign tumors, infections and various anatomic abnormalities. His knowledge extends to the evaluation and treatment of infertility. The obstetrician-gynecologist is particularly knowledgeable about the efficacy and adverse effects of various methods of birth control.

THE AMERICAN BOARD OF OPHTHALMOLOGY

REQUIREMENTS FOR CERTIFICATION
1. Applicant must be a licensed doctor of medicine.
2. Three years of residency and basic science courses in ophthalmology.
3. One year of independent practice or research.
4. Successful completion of a written and oral examination administered by the Board.

SPECIAL SKILLS   The ophthalmologist restricts his practice to the medical and surgical treatment of diseases of the eye. These include, among others, cataracts, glaucoma, injuries, infections and tumors. He has extensive experience in the use of several special instruments to examine the interior of the eye for signs of disease. He has a thorough understanding of the principles of the science of optics and can therefore determine whether and how a particular defect in vision can be corrected by glasses. Finally, he has had extensive training and experience in the complex and delicate surgical treatment of eye diseases.

THE AMERICAN BOARD OF ORTHOPEDIC SURGERY

REQUIREMENTS FOR CERTIFICATION
1. Applicant must be a licensed doctor of medicine.
2. Four years of orthopedic education.
3. One year of independent practice.
4. Successful completion of an examination administered by the Board.

SPECIAL SKILLS The orthopedist specializes in the diagnosis and treatment of diseases of the bones and joints. Most patients think of him primarily as the doctor who knows best how to treat broken bones but this represents only a small fraction of his knowledge and skills. The practice of orthopedics includes the treatment of inherited and infectious diseases of bones and joints which are correctable by surgery. The orthopedist also treats the great variety of bone tumors, and he is particularly expert in hand surgery and back surgery. He can often alleviate the pain and deformity of certain crippling forms of arthritis by appropriate surgical intervention.

Because of his special knowledge of the mechanics of muscular and skeletal function he frequently serves as the physician for amateur and professional athletic teams.

THE AMERICAN BOARD OF OTOLARYNGOLOGY

REQUIREMENTS FOR CERTIFICATION
1. Applicant shall be a licensed doctor of medicine.
2. One year of residency in general surgery.
3. Three years of residency in otolaryngology.
4. Successful completion of oral and written examinations administered by the Board.

SPECIAL SKILLS Otolaryngology, or otorhinolaryngology, is the specialty devoted to the care of patients with diseases of the ear, nose and throat (E.N.T.). The specialist in this area can examine the interior of these organs is great detail with the aid of instruments that permit direct visualization with little discomfort. He can treat both the surgical and the medical disorders peculiar to these structures including, among others, hearing loss, infections, allergies and tumors. He also is frequently called upon by his medical colleagues to surgically insert a tube into a patient's trachea (tracheostomy) as a life-saving procedure when the patient is in severe respiratory distress.

THE SPECIALIST AND WHAT HE CAN DO

THE AMERICAN BOARD OF PATHOLOGY

REQUIREMENTS FOR CERTIFICATION
1. Applicant must be a licensed doctor of medicine or osteopathy.
2. Four years of training in both clinical and anatomic pathology.
3. Or three years of training in either clinical or anatomic pathology.
4. Or eight years of practical experience under circumstances acceptable to the Board.
5. Successful completion of examinations administered by the Board.

SPECIAL SKILLS The patient has little opportunity for personal contact with this specialist but he is a vital member of the health care team. He serves the patient by providing a great number of different laboratory tests for the evaluation of the patient's blood, other body fluids and tissues. This specialty therefore provides other specialists with much of the information which enables them to care for their patients. The pathologist also performs autopsies (postmortem examinations) to help identify the specific diseases responsible for the patient's death. This information often enables the physician to improve his fund of knowledge for the care of future patients. Surely if this specialty didn't exist it would be very difficult to offer the patient many of the benefits of modern medical care.

THE AMERICAN BOARD OF PEDIATRICS

REQUIREMENTS FOR CERTIFICATION IN GENERAL PEDIATRICS
1. The applicant must be a licensed doctor of medicine or osteopathy.
2. A minimum of two years of training in general pediatrics.
3. A minimum of one additional year of training in either general pediatrics, a pediatric subspecialty, or training in another medical field.
4. Two additional years of either further training or independent practice.
5. Successful completion of a written and an oral examination administered by the Board.

REQUIREMENTS FOR CERTIFICATION IN SUBSPECIALTY AREAS
As is the case with Internal Medicine there are a number of subspecialties which fall within the scope of general pediatrics. These include, among others, pediatric cardiology, allergy, hematology, neurology and so forth. Although the training in each of these areas is rigorous and well defined, only pediatric cardiology has its own separate examining board at the present time.

REQUIREMENTS FOR CERTIFICATION IN PEDIATRIC CARDIOLOGY
1. Prior certification in general pediatrics (see above).
2. Two additional years of full-time training.
3. Successful completion of a written and an oral examination by the subspecialty board.

SPECIAL SKILLS   The pediatrician is trained in the diagnosis and treatment of virtually all the diseases of children. His patients include the unborn, the newborn, the teenager, and children of all ages in between. He must, therefore, have as broad an understanding of the diseases of childhood as the internist has of the illnesses of adulthood, many of which are the same. There are, however, many important differences.

The pediatrician has particular expertise in the inheritable diseases and illnesses which afflict the unborn child. He therefore can be extremely useful to prospective parents who may be concerned about the likelihood of future children being affected by various inherited diseases. This function is known as "genetic counseling."

He can learn a great deal about the existence of such diseases in the unborn child by a special procedure called "amniocentesis." In this procedure a needle is inserted through the pregnant mother's abdomen into her uterus (womb) and some of the fluid surrounding the fetus (unborn child) is removed for analysis. Depending on the results of this examination the pediatrician may be in a position to recommend either completion of the pregnancy in a normal fashion, abortion, or treatment of the fetus. The latter may be recommended in cases of "Rh incompatibility," in which the mother's body has the capacity to destroy the fetus's red blood cells. The unborn child can then be given blood transfusions by a process similar to amniocentesis in which the needle is placed into the fetus's abdomen and blood is injected.

After a child is born, the pediatrician is responsible for his care in the hospital. The skill required to do this is especially refined when the newborn child is premature or otherwise seriously ill. Many of these children wouldn't survive if it weren't for the knowledge and care of the well-trained pediatrician.

Most patients are quite familiar with the pediatrician because of the role he plays in the observation of the child's growth and development, nutrition, immunizations and treatment of the common childhood illnesses. These areas can also be handled perfectly adequately by the well trained and experienced family practitioner if the child's parents so choose. The pediatrician, however, is particularly necessary for the proper care of the more serious illnesses of childhood such as certain severe behavior problems, mental retardation, infections, heart diseases, cancers and so forth.

At some point in adolescence the child becomes more susceptible to the diseases of adulthood. The parents and the pediatrician usually recognize when this occurs and they decide that the child should be cared for by another physician, often an internist or a family practitioner. The pediatrician then usually steps aside with the satisfaction that he has helped the youngster get a healthy start in life.

THE AMERICAN BOARD OF PHYSICAL MEDICINE AND REHABILITATION

REQUIREMENTS FOR CERTIFICATION

1. The applicant must be a licensed doctor of medicine.
2. A minimum of three years of postgraduate training, two of which must be specifically devoted to physical medicine and rehabilitation (PMR).
3. Two additional years of full-time independent practice of the specialty.
4. Successful completion of a written and an oral examination administered by the Board.

NOTE: A minimum of eight years of full-time practice of PMR may be an acceptable substitute for requirement #2.

SPECIAL SKILLS The specialist in physical medicine and rehabilitation has the knowledge and ability to assist patients to regain a number of body functions which have been impaired by a wide variety of diseases. Among other things he can help victims of stroke, polio and spinal cord injury to reacquire at least some use of their arms and legs. The stiffness and pain of arthritic joints can be greatly alleviated by his techniques. Many elderly or chronically ill patients who may be bedridden because of weakness and disease of their muscles can be strengthened enough by his exercises to get out of bed and care for themselves.

The techniques employed in this specialty include the medical use of such physical agents as heat, water, electricity and ultraviolet light as well as the use of massage and exercise. The specialist must be familiar with the structure and function of each muscle and joint in order to apply the appropriate form of therapy for each particular condition.

The specialist in PMR is a valuable member of the health care team not only because of the intrinsic importance of his skills but also because most other physicians receive little or no training in this field.

THE AMERICAN BOARD OF PLASTIC SURGERY

REQUIREMENTS FOR CERTIFICATION

1. The applicant must be a licensed doctor of medicine or osteopathy.
2. Three years of training in general surgery or prior certification by any one of several surgical specialty boards.
3. A minimum of two additional years of training in plastic surgery.
4. Successful completion of a written and an oral examination administered by the Board.

SPECIAL SKILLS   Most patients are familiar with the plastic surgeon because of his ability to improve the appearance of certain undesirable facial features such as cleft lip, "hooked" nose or wrinkles. His talents, however, are far from limited to these problems alone. He can surgically correct or modify a great number of inherited and acquired defects and deformities of the face, neck, body and extremities in order to improve function as well as appearance. He is especially qualified to minimize the scarring which frequently results after a serious burn.

THE AMERICAN BOARD OF PREVENTIVE MEDICINE

REQUIREMENTS FOR CERTIFICATION
1. The applicant must be a licensed doctor of medicine or osteopathy.
2. A minimum of three years of specialized training.
3. A minimum of one year of independent research, teaching or practice.
4. Successful completion of a written and an oral examination administered by the Board.

Four general areas are contained within this general category: Public Health, Aerospace Medicine, Occupational Medicine and General Preventive Medicine. The specific requirements for certification vary somewhat for each subspecialty but follow the general outline given above.

SPECIAL SKILLS Relatively few people will ever have a typical patient-doctor relationship with an individual trained in one of these fields of preventive medicine. These specialists are usually involved in administration, teaching or research and see patients only in unusual circumstances.

The specialist in Public Health is concerned with the nonmedical aspects of our society which can have a deleterious effect on large groups of people. In this capacity he is involved in identifying harmful by-products of industry, establishing criteria for the safe handling of food products, and the like. He may investigate epidemics and try to discover trends in the frequency with which certain diseases occur. He is alert to possible environmental factors which may cause or aggravate disease. These functions are usually carried out in a university, in a governmental agency or as a consultant to industry.

Aerospace Medicine, as the name implies, deals with the unique aspects of bodily function under the stress of space flight. Many discoveries made by specialists in this area are finding application to the care of earthbound patients with a number of different diseases. Further discussion of this area of medicine is beyond the scope of this book.

Occupational Medicine is a specialty which studies the particular health hazards associated with various types of work. The specialist is trained to identify and evaluate the harmful aspects of working conditions in many different industries which jeopardize the health of employees. His recommendations are presented to industry and various regulatory agencies so that appropriate corrective action can be undertaken.

The specialist in General Preventive Medicine is qualified to perform many functions in the areas of Public Health and Occupational Medicine.

THE AMERICAN BOARD OF PSYCHIATRY AND NEUROLOGY

This Board certifies that physicians have received adequate training in four areas: psychiatry, neurology, child psychiatry and neurology with special competence in child neurology.

REQUIREMENTS FOR CERTIFICATION

Psychiatry or Neurology
1. The applicant must be a licensed doctor of medicine or osteopathy.
2. Three years of specialized training in either psychiatry or neurology.
3. Two additional years of satisfactory experience in psychiatry or neurology.
4. Successful completion of a written and an oral examination administered by the Board.

Neurology with Special Competence in Child Neurology

1. One year of general pediatric residency.
2. Two years of general neurologic residency.
3. Two or three additional years of training and experience in child neurology.
4. Successful completion of a written and an oral examination administered by the Board.

Child Psychiatry
1. Prior certification by the Board in the area of general psychiatry.
2. Two additional years of training in an approved child psychiatry training program.
3. Successful completion of an examination administered by the Board.

SPECIAL SKILLS   *Psychiatry and Child Psychiatry:* During his training the psychiatrist learns how to detect and treat many of the disorders of the mind and emotions. His special skills include a profound knowledge of human behavior, thought processes and emotions; a thorough knowledge of his own in particular; and the patience, willingness and ability to learn about those peculiar to his patients. He can apply these skills to a particular patient's problem and establish a relationship with him through which the patient is helped to understand his problem and cope with it. In some cases the psychiatrist may use certain drugs to bring about a decrease in a particular distressing symptom such as anxiety or depression which might interfere with successful therapy. Most of us have problems such as these (neuroses) at some point in our lives.

Some patients have much more severe disorders which cause them to lose touch with reality in one way or another (psychoses). The psychiatrist can be of some assistance to these patients by providing them with support during periodic crises and continuing observation and discussion (psychotherapy). Heavy reliance is placed on drugs to help these patients function as normally as possible. These medications are effective in part because of the strong likelihood that many psychiatric disorders are due to chemical imbalances in the brain.

The psychiatrist can also help another group of patients who have structural brain diseases such as stroke, cerebral palsy and so on. Some of these patients become forgetful, overly talkative or mute, and have wide and rapid swings in emotion as well as other symptoms. Some of these patients recognize what has happened to them and become anxious, depressed or paranoid as a result. The psychiatrist can help to control some of these symptoms with appropriate drugs. There is little he or any other physician can do about the underlying disease, however.

The child psychiatrist is skilled in dealing with the psychiatric problems of children. A comprehensive discussion of this area is beyond the scope of this book, but we should mention that this specialist is perhaps the most qualified physician to deal with children who have learning disorders, who are hyperactive and who have serious behavior problems.

Neurology and Child Neurology: These specialists are concerned primarily with diseases of the nervous system (brain, spinal cord and nerves). They possess many skills in common with the neurosurgeon (see above) but they are not qualified to perform surgical operations. The patient with a neurological disease will probably be referred by his internist to a neurologist. After the neurologist evaluates the patient he will either treat him himself or, if the patient needs surgery, he will be referred to a neurosurgeon.

THE AMERICAN BOARD OF RADIOLOGY

REQUIREMENTS FOR CERTIFICATION

There are many subspecialties within the general area of radiology. We shall concern ourselves here with two areas: Diagnostic Radiology and Therapeutic Radiology. Patients will have little contact with specialists in the other areas.

1. The applicant must be a licensed doctor of medicine or osteopathy.
2. Three years of residency training in either diagnostic or therapeutic radiology.
3. One additional year of training in another medical field.
4. Successful completion of a written and an oral examination administered by the Board.

SPECIAL SKILLS *Diagnostic Radiology:* The specialist in diagnostic radiology has been trained to use certain forms of radiant energy (such as x-rays) in order to detect abnormalities in the structure or function of internal organs. Most of us have had chest or bone x-rays which have been interpreted by a diagnostic radiologist. There is a long list of other x-ray procedures which this specialist can perform. Indeed, there is hardly an organ in the body which cannot be visualized by one technique or other. Some of the more common ones include examination of the gallbladder (cholecystography), the esophagus, stomach and duodenum (upper gastrointestinal series), the large bowel (barium enema), to name only a few.

The diagnostic radiologist is also trained in a special field called Nuclear Radiology. This field is somewhat similar to Nuclear Medicine (see above) in that the specialist uses radioactive materials rather than x-rays to visualize various internal organs.

Therapeutic Radiology: This highly specialized field is devoted to the treatment, with high doses of radioactivity, of patients who have some form of cancer. The radioactive energy can be directed specifically to the area of the body which contains the tumor and, in many cases, it causes the tumor to decrease in size or completely disappear.

The therapeutic radiologist must have a thorough knowledge of the many diseases he treats by this method. He must carefully evaluate each patient before therapy begins and at each visit in order to determine the effectiveness of the treatments. He must know exactly how much radiation should be sufficient to produce the best results while causing the least amount of damage to the normal organs near the tumor. He, therefore, must know how much radiation is necessary for the treatment of each kind of tumor as well as the acceptable limits of radioactivity which each normal organ can tolerate. Finally, he must be able to select the kind of radioactive energy which is best suited for the treatment of each case and how to deliver it.

Thanks to the members of this specialty the public has available today a sometimes curative, and frequently helpful, method to treat cancer.

THE AMERICAN BOARD OF SURGERY

REQUIREMENTS FOR CERTIFICATION
1. The applicant must be a licensed doctor of medicine.
2. A minimum of four years of residency training in general surgery.
3. Successful completion of a written and an oral examination administered by the Board.

SPECIAL SKILLS   It is beyond the scope of this book to discuss in detail all of the many skills possessed by a surgeon. In general terms he must be thoroughly familiar with the complex anatomy of the human body. He must understand the normal functions of each organ and how these functions are altered by a huge number of diseases. He must know which diseases can be treated surgically and how and when to operate. He must be skilled in the preparation of patients for surgery and in the care of the patient afterward. He must be aware of the multitude of potential complications of surgery and he must know how to anticipate them and treat them.

The breadth of the knowledge and skills expected of the surgeon can be best summarized by quoting from the requirements listed by the American Board of Surgery: "Candidates for examination are expected to have a detailed knowledge of surgery of the gastrointestinal tract and other abdominal conditions, of the breast and the head and neck. In addition they are expected to possess an adequate breadth and depth of and experience in the management of musculoskeletal trauma and head injuries, and of the more common problems in cardiothoracic, vascular, gynecologic, neurologic, orthopedic, pediatric, plastic and urologic surgery."

THE AMERICAN BOARD OF THORACIC SURGERY

REQUIREMENTS FOR CERTIFICATION
1. Prior certification by the American Board of Surgery.
2. Two additional years of training in thoracic surgery.
3. Successful completion of a written and an oral examination administered by the Board.

SPECIAL SKILLS   The thoracic surgeon is one of the most highly skilled of all medical specialists. He is probably best known for his ability to perform open heart surgery. This procedure requires the use of the "heart-lung" machine which performs the functions of these two organs while the patient is undergoing surgery. During the operation the surgeon attempts to repair one or more structures within the heart such as its valves, its muscle or its blood vessels. The surgeon must be expert in the diagnosis of heart disease. He must know which patients are likely to benefit from surgery and he must decide when the operations should be performed. He must be able to treat immediately the many complications that arise during and after surgery. For this skill alone hundreds of thousands of patients own their lives to the thoracic surgeon.

In some major medical centers these surgeons are able to perform heart transplants. Although this is a controversial area because of many failures, the surgeon has rarely been to blame. The basic problem is that the body mounts its natural defense mechanisms and destroys the transplanted heart. It is up to the immunologists to solve this problem. When it is finally solved, heart transplantation may become a frequently performed, lifesaving surgical procedure.

The thoracic surgeon also operates on the other organs in the chest: notably the lungs (especially for lung cancer), the major blood vessels and the esophagus. Given the incredible responsibility for the life of his patient which the thoracic surgeon accepts each time he operates there is little wonder that the training period is so long and arduous.

THE AMERICAN BOARD OF UROLOGY

REQUIREMENTS FOR CERTIFICATION
1. The applicant must be a licensed doctor of medicine.
2. Two years of training in general surgery.
3. Three additional years of training in urologic surgery.
4. Eighteen months of independent practice.
5. Successful completion of a written and an oral examination administered by the Board.

SPECIAL SKILLS The urologist restricts his practice to those diseases which affect the kidneys, urinary bladder, prostate gland and male sex organs. He is highly skilled in a number of x-ray techniques (e.g., intravenous pyelography, IVP) which permit clear visualization of the kidneys, the bladder and the tubes which connect them (the ureters). He can see into the inside of the urinary bladder and visualize part of the prostate gland with the aid of an instrument called a cystoscope.

He is a surgeon and as such can operate on these organs to repair hereditary defects, to drain abscesses, to remove stones and to treat cancer. Much of his time is spent removing part or all of the prostate gland which enlarges with age and can block the normal flow of urine out of the bladder in older men.

Other skills include expert surgical treatment of cancer of the testicle, performance of vasectomy to produce male sterilization, and he is an essential member of the kidney transplant team.

5

What You Should Know About Your Local Hospital

THE HOSPITAL TODAY is the cornerstone of the health care delivery system. Within its walls a vast array of services are distributed to both sick and healthy members of society in order to restore and maintain their health. Even the smallest hospital is a highly complex institution which coordinates the professional activities of physicians, nurses, social workers, technologists, nutritionists, administrators and support personnel. Because it brings together the services of all these health care professionals, the hospital is particularly suited for the management of serious, puzzling and complicated illnesses.

WHAT TYPES OF HOSPITAL ARE AVAILABLE IN YOUR COMMUNITY?

Just as your needs for a physician vary from one time to another so do your requirements of a hospital. An acute care general hospital can provide adequate services for most common illnesses. When major debilitating or life-threatening illnesses such as cancer or kidney failure strike, or when you need sophisticated surgical procedures such as open heart surgery or neurosurgery, you will usually get better care in a specialized medical center or university hospital, where the equipment and personnel experienced in managing these illnesses are located.

The American Hospital Association publishes a book entitled *The AHA Guide to the Health Care Field*, which provides a great deal of helpful information about individual hospitals throughout the country. Information which is of special concern to the consumer includes selected services and facilities available, whether the hospital is eligible for payments by Medicaid, Medicare, Blue Cross and other third party payers and whether the hospital is accredited by the Joint Commission on Accreditation of Hospitals (see below). We recommend that you refer to this book, which should be available in your public library.

Hospitals may be classified according to *function* and in terms of *ownership* or *financial support*.

FUNCTION *Acute Care Hospitals:* The hospital found in most communities usually falls under this heading. It is oriented, designed, equipped and staffed to take care of patients with acute illnesses or flare-ups of chronic illnesses. The average length of stay is usually relatively short, on the order of seven to ten days. The scope of services it provides depends on the size of the community in which it is located and whether or not it is affiliated with a medical school or reseach foundation. For example, the acute care hospital in a suburban or rural community is likely to be able to care for most common illnesses but may not be equipped or staffed for open heart surgery, kidney transplantation, cancer therapy and the like.

You would be wise, therefore, if you already know you have a major and complicated illness, to find out whether your local hospital can provide you with the care you may need. A direct question in this regard to your doctor or the hospital administrator should settle the matter. If it is not adequate for your specialized needs, you should ask your doctor to refer you to a specialist who is affiliated with a hospital that is, even if he and it are many miles away. The benefits you stand to derive in this fashion far outweigh the inconvenience of a long drive.

Chronic Disease Hospitals: These hospitals are particularly suited for the care of patients with a variety of orthopedic, neuromuscular, neurological and mental illnesses who require custodial care, physical and occupational therapy and the regular attention of a physician.

Special Disease Hospitals: Usually, but not invariably, affiliated with a medical school or research foundation, these hospitals restrict their services to patients with a selected disease or group of diseases. Because of this degree of specialization the hospitals are usually equipped with the most modern equipment necesary to deal with these diseases. The physicians are highly skilled in diagnosis, management and treatment, and the nurses are experienced in caring for the particular needs of the patients hospitalized therein. Hospitals of this sort exist for the treatment of cancer, bone and joint diseases, eye diseases, burns, muscle diseases, diseases of children, disorders peculiar to childbearing, and so on.

If you now have or develop one of these problems in the future and neither your physician nor your local hospital are particularly experienced or equipped to deal with it you should make every effort to be evaluated by a specialist at one of these hospitals if at all possible. Frequently only a few visits are necessary during which an expert diagnosis can be made. The specialist can then advise your local physician how to best treat your illness and you can return home. Sometimes, however, the equipment necessary for treatment is so new and expensive that it is only available at one of these centers and you may have to remain there or return periodically for treatment. In any event these specialized centers fill a great need in our society and should be utilized thoroughly to supplement generally available facilities.

OWNERSHIP Hospitals can be classified also according to ownership or primary source of financial support.

Government Supported Hospitals: These include military, Veterans Administration, Public Health Service, state, county and city hospitals. They are tax-supported and medical care is provided free of charge to qualified patients. You must meet certain minimal requirements in order to qualify for admission to these facilities; so if they are available in your area find out if you are eligible by simply phoning the administrator's office. Many of these hospitals are affiliated with medical schools and postgraduate medical training programs and provide very high quality medical care.

Nonprofit Hospitals: These hospitals are dependent on contributions, endowments and patients' fees for their support. They are often sponsored by religious groups and many are closely affiliated with medical schools and research foundations. They are most commonly acute care facilities but many restrict their services to patients with selected diseases. The range of services available varies according to a number of factors mentioned above but generally excellent care is provided. The continuous, around the clock presence of interns and residents in those hospitals affiliated with universities is highly desirable for obvious reasons and the very fact that they are training centers generally assures you that the full-time staff physicians have been selected for their demonstrated awareness of modern medical advances and ability to apply this knowledge to the analysis and management of difficult cases.

Proprietary Hospitals: These facilities are usually operated for a profit and are owned by individuals or stockholders many of whom may be the same physicians who admit their own private patients to the hospital. The potential for conflict of interest is obvious. The medical services available in these hospitals are frequently more limited than those found in voluntary nonprofit hospitals but many excellent proprietary hospitals can nevertheless be found.

In brief, in choosing the general type of hospital most suited to your needs at any given time you should ask yourself the following questions:

1. "Am I Likely to Require the Services of an Acute Care, Chronic Disease or Specialized Hospital or a Combination of These?"

We reiterate that most problems can be handled by acute care hospitals, especially those which are affiliated with universities or research foundations. Since it is usually more desirable, however, to be hospitalized locally and because university-affiliated teaching hospitals have only a limited number of beds, you should use the local facility for most purposes. You can get some idea of its capabilities by asking for a copy of the hospital's annual report which should list the names and specialties of the staff physicians, the number of patients seen, the special procedures which were performed and the like. If you have cancer or a major illness for which a cancer center or otherwise specialized hospital is available you should make every effort to have your case reviewed by their staff and perhaps even go there for care. Although highly competent physicians in these fields are frequently available in local communities there is no question that, by and large, more thorough and critical evaluation is possible at these specialized centers.

2. "Does My Physician Have Admitting Privileges at One or More of these Hospitals?"

No matter how good the hospitals in your community are it may be difficult to derive the greatest benefit from them unless your personal physician is on the staff. Make sure your doctor is on the staff of at least one good hospital. Except in very unusual circumstances the doctor without admitting privileges has chosen to confine his practice to only minor or otherwise restricted problems or has been refused these privileges by the hospitals for some reason. In either event he will not be able to provide continuing care through a period of hospitalization when you may need him most.

3. "Am I Eligible for Hospitalization in a Government Subsidized Facility?"

If you are a veteran check with your local Veterans Administration information officer. For information about state or local governmental hospitals call them directly and speak with the patients' affairs representative or social worker.

4. "Is the Hospital of My Choice Approved by the Joint Commission on Accreditation of Hospitals?"

This commission is composed of representatives from the following organizations: The American College of Surgeons, The American College of Physicians, The American Hospital Association, The American Medical Association and The Canadian Medical Association. Its function is to establish the *minimum* standards which hospitals must meet in order to provide an acceptable (not superior) level of medical care; to inspect hospitals every three years to determine whether these standards are being fulfilled; and to award a certificate of accreditation to those hospitals which are approved. This certificate is usually displayed in some prominent public location (usually the lobby) in approved hospitals. Only approved hospitals are eligible to participate in the Medicare program and to receive governmental funds for the support of training programs for interns, residents, nurses and so on. Approval by the JCAH should therefore be one of your absolute requirements in the selection of a hospital.

WHAT ARE THE ESSENTIAL FEATURES OF A MODERN ACUTE CARE HOSPITAL?

If you have decided that your needs will be best served in an acute care hospital, there are several criteria available whereby you can evaluate how well a given hospital fits your particular needs.

What Kinds of Doctors Are on the Staff?

Naturally, the wider the variety of medical and surgical specialists on the staff of a hospital, the more comprehensive will the services be that it can provide to the patient. Generally speaking, a specialist will not even apply for staff privileges at a hospital unless it has or promises to obtain the equipment and support personnel necessary for him to practice his specialty. The presence of many different specialists as well as general physicians therefore increases the likelihood that a particular hospital will be able to serve you in most clinical situations.

The presence of many board certified specialists also provides you with reasonable assurances that high quality medicine is being practiced by all members of the group. The reason for this is that the more training a doctor gets the more he is likely to realize how little he really knows. He therefore is not ashamed to refer his patients to other doctors more knowledgeable than he is in a particular area. The whole environment is conducive to communication, education, and free interchange of ideas. Furthermore, every doctor's methods are visible to all of the other doctors. The peer pressure that results from this kind of professional exposure provides additional impetus for the doctor to remain abreast of developments in his field.

How Well Trained Are the Nurses?

There are three general categories into which nursing personnel may fall:

THE REGISTERED NURSE (RN) has had the most extensive professional education and has completed between three and five years of training after high school. Some RN's also have a bachelor's degree in nursing which they have earned by completing a full college curriculum as well as their professional nursing training. After passing a licensure examination the nurse receives the "RN" designation and earns the right to supervise and coordinate the nursing activities on a hospital ward, in an outpatient clinic or the like.

THE LICENSED VOCATIONAL (PRACTICAL) NURSE (LVN OR LPN) has had a one year training program after high school and has passed a licensure examination. These nurses can perform most of the duties of the RN but are not permitted to act in a supervisory or administrative capacity. They are extremely important for the day-to-day care of the patient and the smooth functioning of the health care delivery unit.

THE NURSING ATTENDANT (NURSES' AIDE) may or may not have completed a six-to-ten weeks on-the-job course. A high school diploma is not required but it is preferred. Most of the duties necessary for the personal needs and comfort of the patient are provided by the Nurses' Aide. Specific medical duties like changing dressings, giving medicines and other professional services must be provided, however, by an RN or LVN.

When you are evaluating a hospital, therefore, be sure to check the annual report to find out the relative distribution of nursing personnel in these three categories. There should be a balance, and most hospitals will have fewer RN's than LVN's and fewer LVN's than Nurses'

Aides. In most hospitals there should be at least two RN's on duty on every ward during all three shifts, and preferably more during the busy day shift. An absolute minimum of one RN and one LVN should be present even during the night shift when things are generally quiet. Emergencies which require the full attention of at least one nurse can occur at any time. The hospital should anticipate this situation and have at least two qualified nurses on duty at all times so that one can be free to care for the remaining patients while the other is fully occupied with an emergency.

What Kinds of Support Personnel Are Available?

Although physical and occupational therapists are important members of the health care team and should be on the staff of all but the smallest acute care hospitals, their services are rarely needed in emergency situations. On the other hand, the services of the respiratory therapist and blood bank technologist should be available around the clock. Find out if personnel trained in these areas are employed by the hospital, especially if you already know that you have a serious lung disease such as emphysema or a bleeding disorder such as hemophilia. Your life may depend on the availability and experience of these technologists so it would be wise to find out if they are employed by the hospital and how available they are after 5 or 6 P.M.

Are There Doctors Present in the Hospital around the Clock?

In many small community hospitals that don't have active teaching programs there aren't any physicians routinely present in the hospital during the night. Since life-threatening emergencies occur regardless of the time of day it is obviously desirable to have a licensed physician on the premises at all times. Some local hospitals solve this problem by hiring off-duty residents from nearby university hospitals to work in the hospital during these nighttime hours. If your local hospital doesn't have twenty-four-hour-a-day coverage we strongly advise that you urge the hospital administration to correct this situation.

Are There Facilities and Personnel Trained in the Delivery of Intensive Care?

Medical science and technology have advanced to the stage where many lives can be saved by the application of modern principles of intensive care medicine. Such services can be provided efficiently only in a special unit designed specifically to accommodate the necessary equipment: an Intensive Care Unit. The vital functions of the patients with a variety of life-threatening illnesses such as heart attack, massive hemorrhage, coma, respiratory failure, kidney failure and many complications of surgery can be constantly monitored and highly complicated, and individualized treatment can be administered in such units. We therefore recommend that if possible you should select a doctor who is on the staff of a hospital that has such a unit. If none exists in your community it will be worth the effort to apply public pressure on the hospital administration to raise the funds necessary to establish one.

Is There an "Emergency Cart" on Each Hospital Ward?

Every hospital ward should be equipped with an emergency cart supplied with the drugs and materials necessary for cardiopulmonary resuscitation. Cardiac arrest and respiratory failure can occur suddenly and unexpectedly in patients hospitalized for nonemergency indications on general hospital floors. These patients stand little chance for survival if cardiac or respiratory arrest develops and the hospital staff is not prepared to treat it immediately. An appropriately equipped emergency cart properly used by trained personnel can often make the difference between life and death.

Is There an Emergency Room on the Premises and How Is It Staffed?

See Chapter 6 for a discussion of emergency care.

What Are the Capabilities of the Diagnostic Laboratory?

There is no question that the overall quality of medical care delivered by a modern hospital today is limited by the quality of services available from the diagnostic laboratory. The laboratory is usually organized by a pathologist. It is his responsibility to supervise the examination of all materials obtained from the patient such as blood, urine, feces, body fluids and tissues removed at surgery or by biopsy techniques. Your doctor makes major decisions regarding your health care based on the reports he gets from the pathologist. Although it is beyond the scope of this book to analyze the importance of each laboratory procedure, there are certain areas which are absolutely critical to the well-being of the patient:

Blood Bank

Careful, accurate and rapid service from the blood bank is essential and may be lifesaving when large amounts of blood must be administered in a hurry. On the other hand, a mistake in determining the patient's blood type may result in a mismatched transfusion followed by a life-threatening transfusion reaction. The blood bank must be carefully supervised and staffed only by specially trained personnel.

"Stat" Lab

This is a slang term for those services which should be provided by the laboratory to the physician in emergency situations. There are a limited number of tests that fall into this category. The results should be available within a short period of time and their accuracy must be without question because life and death decisions frequently depend on them.

Surgical Pathology Service

When tissue is removed from the body at surgery or by a biopsy procedure it is sent to the surgical pathology laboratory, where it is examined by the pathologist. Decisions regarding the nature of the disease present in the tissue and whether or not it is cancer depend on the pathologist's subjective interpretation. The importance of a highly trained and experienced pathologist under these circumstances should be obvious. Since no pathologist can be expert in more than a few areas of tissue pathology it is frequently necessary to send the tissue or slides to experts at larger institutions for consultation. Therefore, if you have a puzzling or serious illness and the question of cancer comes up based on the interpretation of a single pathologist working alone in a small community hospital, you should insist that the slides or tissue be sent to other pathologists for confirmation. This amounts to no more than good medical practice. It is the only logical thing to do.

Due to its complexity and because virtually all of its services are delivered by fallible human beings, errors will inevitably occur in even the finest of hospitals despite the strictest of safeguards. A generous and understanding attitude on the part of the consumer is warranted under most of these circumstances if your hospital meets the standards outlined in this chapter. If it lacks adequate equipment and personnel we strongly encourage you to exert public pressure on the hospital board of trustees to rectify the situation. After all, it is your life that hangs in the balance.

6

Emergency Medical Care

A WELL-EQUIPPED and properly staffed hospital emergency room (ER) is, no doubt, the best place to go for emergency medical care and among the worst for minor and chronic illnesses. In order to derive the greatest possible benefit from a visit to the emergency room, the consumer must know considerably more than simply how to get there.

WHAT CONSTITUTES A TRUE EMERGENCY?

One of the commonest reasons for consumer dissatisfaction with emergency care stems from the inappropriate use of the ER (Emergency Room) by the public for the care of nonemergency ailments. This causes crowding and confusion with all of the accompanying delays and aggravation. The ER staff must then either see patients in the order of their arrival regardless of the nature of the problem or assign priority ratings to patients according to the urgency of their ailment. The latter method is immensely preferable but it requires the attendance of a medically trained screening officer whose talents would be better employed in the actual care of patients. Both methods are costly and the costs are naturally borne by the consumer. The pity is that such screening personnel would be largely unnecessary if only patients with truly urgent problems came to the ER for care.

How, then, can you recognize what constitutes a true emergency? Most major emergencies are obvious and fall into several distinct categories:

1. Sudden, unexplained and unexpected onset of severe pain in the chest, abdomen, head, neck and back.
2. Loss of large amounts of blood in vomitus, diarrhea, urine, or from the vagina.
3. Loss of consciousness or sudden impairment of mental function.
4. Prolonged convulsions.
5. Sudden or severe difficulty in breathing.
6. Sudden and severe impairment of vision or chemical and mechanical injury to the eye.
7. Major burns.
8. Fractured bones.

9. Skull and spine injuries.
10. Gunshot and knife wounds and other life-threatening injuries.
11. Serious lacerations.
12. Ingestion of potentially poisonous substances.
13. Severe, incapacitating psychiatric decompensation.
14. Poisonous snake and insect bites.

The above listed situations obviously require *emergency* medical care which can be rendered most efficiently in a hospital emergency room. There are many other situations, however, which should receive *prompt* attention and can usually be handled adequately in the general physician's office. If your doctor is unavailable, however, or if you aren't quite sure about the urgency of the situation and want professional advice you should call your local ER, explain the situation to the nurse and ask to speak to the doctor on call. They are trained in emergency care and will be able to assess the problem and advise you of its urgency at which time you can decide whether to go to the ER or wait to see your physician in his office.

WHAT SHOULD YOU DO IN THE WAKE OF AN EMERGENCY?

The effective application of a few basic principles of first aid by people at the scene of an emergency can and does save countless lives each year. The prime objectives of emergency care are to preserve the life of the patient and the function of his organs. The prime admonition to those who provide this care is "First, do no harm."

Because the potential benefits from the proper delivery of emergency care are so great and because the consequences of improper care are so dire we strongly recommend that *each and every adult in your household should be properly trained in the delivery of emergency first aid*. Such training is available from a number of sources which vary from community to community. Some courses are given by local chapters of the Red Cross, others by local medical societies, the police and fire departments, or by your local hospital. If none is available in your area you should petition these agencies to offer one or travel to a neighboring community where it may be available. *It is worth all that effort* as anyone whose life has been saved by a passerby or, in contrast, as anyone who is a paraplegic because of careless transportation methods can attest.

We will not discuss the principles and application of emergency first aid in depth in this book. We believe that such information can only be properly obtained in person from trained professionals with the opportunity for supervised practice of your newly acquired skills. Furthermore, the fact that you have read about such methods can lull you into thinking that you know how to apply them. The topics that should be covered in such a course and with which you should be thoroughly familiar are:

1. How to control massive hemorrhage.
2. How to ensure adequate breathing.
3. How to improve blood circulation.
4. How to administer cardiorespiratory resuscitation.
5. What to do after accidental poisoning.
6. How to protect a broken limb.
7. How to prevent spinal cord injury when moving the injured patient.

Mostly what you will learn in such a course is how and why to apply commonsense principles to emergency medical situations. You should also have the chance to practice them under supervision. In the process you will become psychologically more able to act in an emergency. You will also automatically learn how to deal with the common minor emergencies that occur at least once a week in most families with growing children.

There is nothing difficult about emergency first aid and it can be learned by anyone with average intelligence. It does, however, require some effort on your part. One of the major points that we hope to emphasize in this book is that *you can improve the quality of the medical care you and your family receive if you work at it*. No one is going to do it for you. It can't be guaranteed by paying high fees to fancy doctors with plush offices. It can't be enforced by governmental regulation. In sum, if you want it you've got to work to get it; and it can be achieved.

There are a number of other simple things you can do to ensure efficient use of the emergency room facilities and personnel:

1. If there is time, phone the ER before you go there and tell them what has happened. In this way they will know what to expect and can be prepared to treat the problem as soon as you arrive.
2. If the problem is accidental poisoning, drug overdose or a chemical burn, take the bottle or container with you so the doctor will know exactly what he has to treat.
3. If a part of the body has been accidentally amputated take it to be the hospital. Most attempts to rejoin the limb to the body have failed but enough have succeeded to make it worthwhile to try.
4. If you have been bitten by a dog or snake or other animal try to identify it so that appropriate medication or vaccination can be started.
5. Carry, at all times, an identification card listing your blood type, allergies, chronic illnesses and medications. This information can be of great assistance to the doctor and may help him to arrive at a diagnosis and begin treatment much more rapidly than would be possible without it, especially if you are unconscious.
6. Keep a list of emergency phone numbers posted next to your telephone. They should include your doctor, the emergency room, the ambulance service and the regional Poison Control Center. The latter is an agency which can advise you about a nearly endless list of dangerous chemicals; it is staffed around the clock in most areas and should be listed in your local telephone directory. If it isn't, you should be able to get the telephone number from your local hospital. In some large cities there is an "Emergency" Operator (911) who will direct your call to the appropriate agency, but this is not a nationwide service.

HOW SHOULD YOU GET TO THE EMERGENCY ROOM?

Most people can be safely transported to the ER by private car if someone properly trained in emergency first aid is in attendance. The care that can be provided by a properly trained commercial or municipal rescue squad is of great value and may be lifesaving in many cases. These units are usually staffed by former military corpsmen or specially trained medical assistants who can monitor vital life functions and administer oxygen, fluids and drugs under the supervision of a physician in the emergency room via telephone communications.

In some communities these teams have evolved into Mobile Coronary Care Units (MCCU). The MCCU is usually a large van which is fully equipped for the emergency care of heart attack victims and may be staffed either by physicians or specially trained paramedical personnel. They are usually dispatched by one of the local hospitals.

Such rescue squads and MCCU's should be used to care for and transport patients suffering from major, catastrophic emergencies such as life threatening hemorrhage, heart attack and cardiorespiratory arrest. They probably should not be summoned for lesser situations to ensure that they will be immediately available to serve in the most urgent cases.

There are also a variety of situations which are not urgent enough to warrant calling these highly trained emergency units but which are sufficiently complicated or serious to deserve transportation by ambulance. Find out what services are available in your community. Then phone or visit their headquarters and find out what they are qualified to do, the size of their staff, the number of vehicles available and the average time required for them to respond to a call for help. You should then decide, with their help and suggestions, the situations in which each service is most useful and the cases which you can safely transport to the ER yourself. It would then be advisable to make a list of the available emergency transport services in your community and post it next to your telephone with their phone numbers and the situations in which each is most useful. Such a list can be invaluable during an emergency, when most people aren't known for their clearheaded thinking. It should again be apparent that the effort you put into this project will be generously rewarded when you are faced with an emergency situation.

WHAT TO EXPECT WHEN YOU ARRIVE AT THE EMERGENCY ROOM

Depending on the urgency of your problem, the time of day and the type of hospital in which it is located, the emergency room can be a beehive of activity and confusion, an efficient and friendly haven for the acutely ill, or a cold, indifferent and sluggish machine for processing human bodies. In any case you will meet a special group of people and may have to endure certain inconveniences.

A visit to a small town hospital emergency room will probably be pleasant and involve few delays. But highly sophisticated and specialized medical care is less likely to be available in that setting than in a big city municipal or university hospital ER. In contrast, the large, urban emergency room can be an impersonal place with long lines and no privacy. Certainly neither of these stereotypes is universal and most unpleasant experiences are due to administrative inefficiencies. Some of these problems are also generated by the inappropriate use of the emergency room as a family doctor substitute by the public. In any event the hospital emergency room plays a major and important role in the delivery of specialized medical care and it is far and away the best place to go for the care of urgent medical problems.

PERSONNEL

Clerical: Unless the urgency of your problem is overwhelming you will probably have to speak with an admissions clerk before you can see the doctor. You will be asked a number of questions which may seem trivial in comparison with your desire to see a doctor immediately. You can save yourself a lot of time and aggravation if you resign yourself to this ritual. You will be asked for your Social Security number and the name of your health insurance carrier and your policy number, so be sure to carry this information in your wallet at all times. It's a good idea to be accompanied by a relative or friend, if possible, so that he or she can handle this interview for you while you are being examined.

Medical: Your family or personal physician may meet you in the ER or you may see either someone he designates or whoever happens to be on call at the time for emergency room duty. In community hospitals the doctor on call may be a fully trained specialist in emergency medicine who, together with a number of partners, covers the ER twenty-four hours a day. He may be any one of the hospital's general staff physicians who is rotating through an ER call schedule but who is not physically present in the ER at all times. Finally, he may be one of the residents in training at a local university or military hospital who is moonlighting in the community hospital ER in his spare time. These latter doctors are generally quite proficient in this field since they also staff the ER at the university hospitals and must deal with emergencies on a daily basis among their many seriously ill hospitalized patients.

The emergency room nurse is really the central figure who is responsible for keeping the ER functioning smoothly and properly supplied with drugs, dressings and assorted medical paraphernalia. The nurse assists the doctor with most of his procedures and performs a wide variety of routine and emergency nursing chores. He or she usually deserves most of the credit when the ER is functioning well and much of the blame when it isn't.

Paramedical: Many ERs now employ medical assistants who assist in the care of many patients and who are trained and qualified to manage a variety of situations with very little supervision. They are full members of the health care team and can be trusted to perform well and to know their own limitations. There is also an array of other people such as laboratory and x-ray technicians, the quality of whose work has an important impact on the quality of the medical care you receive. Because they are less visible to the patient he is not likely to appreciate how important they are.

STANDARD OPERATING PROCEDURE IN THE EMERGENCY ROOM

If you go to an emergency room for one of the major and urgent problems listed early in this chapter you will probably be seen by a doctor immediately and his evaluation and disposition of your case will be as prompt as possible. On the other hand if you visit the ER for one of the less urgent or nonurgent problems discussed above you may find yourself waiting for long periods while other more urgent cases are given priority. You may have to wait to see the nurse, wait to see the doctor, wait to have lab tests done, wait to have x-rays taken, wait to be seen by a consultant, wait for treatment and wait to be released.

While it is appalling that this happens, hard decisions

concerning priorities have to be made in the ER and the nonurgent case is definitely a low priority. As we mentioned above there are a large number of legitimate semi-urgent situations which require emergency room care. These, however, sometimes cannot be easily distinguished by the clerk from the absolutely nonurgent category and may be lumped together with them and put at the bottom of the waiting list. That is one reason why it is worthwhile to call the ER for advice about these semi-urgent problems. If the physician or nurse instructed you to come in you should announce that fact along with the physician's or nurse's name in a loud and clear voice to the clerk. Such an approach frequently shortens the waiting time considerably.

HOW TO PREPARE FOR EMERGENCIES BEFORE THEY OCCUR

You can do a number of things today which will greatly increase the ease of obtaining prompt medical care when an emergency arises.

1. Have those phone numbers (ambulance, hospital, emergency room, doctors, etc.) we mentioned earlier posted right next to the telephone.
2. Always carry the medical ID card we discussed above (and see Appendix) listing your blood type, allergies, medications, chronic illnesses and immunization record

(especially tetanus toxoid). A card containing this information plus a fairly thorough medical history on microfilm can be obtained from a firm named Emergency Medical Record, 2640 Northaven Road, Suite 107, Dallas, Texas 75229. Alternatively, if you have a major illness or allergy you should consider purchasing one of the medical information bracelets available at most drugstores.

3. If your child is injured or needs emergency care for some other reason while at school or with a baby-sitter most hospitals will not treat him until you have been contacted and have given permission for treatment. It might be wise, therefore, to visit the emergency room in your community and sign a release which gives them permission to treat him even if you can't be reached.

4. Keep a bottle of ipecac at home at all times. This is a drug which induces vomiting when taken by mouth and it is available without a prescription at your drugstore. It is generally used to produce vomiting in children who have accidentally swallowed poisonous substances. *Check with your doctor or emergency room before giving it to your child since it should not be used after swallowing certain caustic agents. Keep it out of your child's reach.*

5. If you or a member of your family are known to have a major illness or allergy you should have your doctor explain whether these conditions are likely to require urgent medical attention in the future. You should also learn specifically what you should do in such an emergency and obtain any necessary equipment or medication which might be needed. If the emergency subsequently occurs you will be prepared to start treatment under your doctor's guidance even before the ambulance arrives.

6. Learn as much as you can about emergency first aid as we discussed above. If no course is available you should read one of the books on the subject and obtain a first aid chart which should be hung in an easily accessible place.
7. Visit the emergency rooms in your community and talk with the head nurse; however, try to avoid particularly busy times in the day such as 7 to 9 A.M. and 3 to 7 P.M., when traffic is heavy. Also avoid holidays and weekends, when emergencies are usually excessive. Inquire about the physicians who staff it, their availability and promptness to respond when needed. Ask about the availability of consultants to the doctor on call, especially anesthesiologists, cardiologists and surgeons. Rank the ERs in order of preference. Although in life-threatening emergencies you should go to the closest emergency room available, in many situations it is safe to drive for a few extra minutes to get to the ER of your choice.

The urgent medical or surgical problem which requires emergency attention is different from the chronic illness in one very important aspect. The patient with the chronic illness can only improve his chances of recovery by selecting the best doctor available and by following his advice. The patient in the emergency situation, however, can greatly influence his chances of survival and recovery by educating himself and his family in the basic principles of emergency care, by being prepared for urgent situations and by knowing precisely how to get assistance and get it fast. If you are willing, therefore, to prepare yourself for such an event your efforts may mean the difference between life and death.

7

Medical Services Available from Community Health Agencies

A LARGE NUMBER of voluntary health organizations offer advice and service to the consumer. Some individuals are even eligible for financial aid from these agencies. Some agencies assist selected patients by providing nursing and homemaker services, hot meals and transportation to and from hospitals and clinics. Others provide educational material about a wide variety of illnesses and distribute newsletters and other bulletins describing medical appliances which may help the handicapped patient in the practical chores of daily living. Some also supply research funds to scientists specifically aimed at discovering the cause, mechanisms and cure for many diseases. This chapter will describe many of these services and agencies and relate their objectives to the specific needs of the consumer-patient.

Local Health Services

In most metropolitan areas and in many suburban and rural communities the following local health services are available:

VISITING NURSE ASSOCIATION

This is usually a community-sponsored program and may be a component of city, county or state public health agencies. The Visiting Nurse makes house calls and provides many health care services such as: wound and bandage care, injections, blood pressure checks, physical therapy, bathing, colostomy and catheter care, etc. The Visiting Nurse also follows a patient's progress and notifies the doctor if any alarming changes occur. Thanks to this service many patients can be discharged earlier from hospitals and others can be kept out of nursing homes.

Some doctors don't make optimal use of the Visiting Nurses Association (VNA). If you or a loved one have a chronic debilitating illness and are hospitalized for prolonged nursing care be sure to remind your doctor of the VNA. Under the proper circumstances hospital time can be shortened, convalescent care facilities can be avoided, money can be saved and the patient can be sent home to be followed by the VNA.

HOME HEALTH AIDES

Some Visiting Nurse Associations and a variety of other community-sponsored and private organizations provide homemaker assistance to the chronically ill or convalescent patient. In fact, there are over 2,300 such agencies throughout the country whose objective is to help care for patients in their homes. The services available from Home Health Aides include such things as shopping, cleaning, preparation of meals and other daily chores necessary to keep a household in order.

The combined benefits available to the public from these two services should be obvious. For example, the ailing mother with a young family can often return home to her children without having to be strong enough to perform housework. The elderly man with a terminal malignancy can be among his loved ones and in familiar surroundings during his final days. The child with a serious illness can often be discharged and return home to be with his brothers, sisters and parents because a Visiting Nurse will come by frequently to check on progress, change his dressings, or give him injections. Large financial savings are also possible if these inexpensive services are utilized because the cost of prolonged confinement in a hospital or nursing home can be eliminated.

MEALS-ON-WHEELS

This is also a community-based service which is usually staffed by volunteers. The major objective of this organization is to provide a balanced diet to housebound patients who are unable to prepare their own meals. Most of the recipients of this service are senior citizens who, without Meals-on-Wheels, would be confined to a nursing home. Usually a hot meal is delivered around lunchtime along with a sandwich, fruit and dessert which can be refrigerated and eaten later in the day.

Many Meals-on-Wheels chapters are affiliated with Senior Citizen Centers. These are frequently located in otherwise unused rooms in local schools, churches or other community based institutions. A hot noonday meal is often provided at the Senior Citizen Center for those people who are well enough to get there on their own or who wish to be transported from home to the center by a community sponsored van. These centers provide a great opportunity for the elderly to get out of their homes and into a social setting. Frequently volunteers teach arts and crafts courses. The conversation is usually lively, and lasting friendships are often formed. The van also may take patients to and from their doctors' offices and is sometimes used for shopping and field trips. The cost for all these services is usually minimal and on a pay-as-you-can basis.

DEPARTMENT OF PUBLIC HEALTH

The Department of Public Health (DPH) is a tax-supported agency which is staffed by physicians, public health nurses, laboratory and x-ray technicians, sanitary inspectors, health educators and supporting personnel. DPH-sponsored clinics usually provide the following services: prenatal care, venereal disease detection and treatment, immunizations, periodic mobile chest x-ray and other screening examinations.

Many other specific services are available to the individual patient but vary from community to community. It would be wise, therefore, to contact your local DPH when you are in need of assistance with medical problems and find out if services tailored to your need are provided.

MEDICAL SUPPLY RENTAL SERVICES

In most metropolitan areas there are private companies that rent such items as hospital beds, wheelchairs and other home care equipment. The availability of these appliances is another force which makes home health care possible and less expensive than hospitalization.

HEALTH AND MEDICAL INFORMATION BY TELEPHONE

In some communities the medical society and other health-oriented agencies have recorded much useful and practical medical information on tape. Individual recordings will be played at your request over the telephone. This is a valuable educational service which can teach the interested caller about the signs, symptoms and ways to prevent many diseases. Check your Yellow Pages for further assistance.

CONSUMER MEDICAL EDUCATION ON TELEVISION

Several programs ("Today's Health," "Feelin' Good") which discuss major health topics in easily understood terms are telecast frequently in many communities. Check your local listings for time and station.

National Voluntary Health Associations

Some of the greatest sources of information and service for patients and their families are the National Voluntary Health Associations which usually have local affiliates in most communities throughout the country.

Over the years we have established professional relationships with local affiliates of many of these agencies and we have been repeatedly impressed by the breadth and depth and practical utility of their patient-oriented programs. We have also been impressed by how many patients and doctors are unaware of the specific services available from these agencies.

We have written this section because of our conviction that greater utilization of these associations by patients and practicing physicians will improve the quality of medical care and expand the services available to the individual. We obtained our information in the following manner. The American Medical Association publishes a directory of National Voluntary Health Organizations which "describes the purpose, organizational pattern, financing and programs of the various national health agencies and other organizations of medical interest . . . based on data submitted by the agencies requesting inclusion in the Directory." Using this list we wrote to each of the agencies and asked them to send us a resume of the services they provide to patients. In most cases we received a prompt and thorough reply. Occasionally our letter was returned by the post office because the addressee had moved and the letter was not forwardable. Rarely, we received no reply at all.

We have carefully reviewed the literature sent to us by these agencies. From this literature we have determined which of these voluntary health agencies actually provide services directly to individual patients. This subgroup of agencies will be considered in the remainder of this chapter. The information provided has been abstracted from the literature supplied by each agency and supplemented by the AMA directory of National Voluntary Health Organizations where necessary.

In addition to these unique and specific services there are a number of general areas in which most organizations resemble one another. We will discuss these general topics first.

OVERALL STRUCTURE AND GENERAL PURPOSE

As defined by the American Medical Association, voluntary health organizations are "non-profit associations of lay and professional persons dedicated to the prevention, alleviation and cure of a particular disease, disability or group of diseases and disabilities."

SUPPORT

The organizations derive the funds necessary to operate from public contributions and also from institutional and governmental sources.

OBJECTIVES

Usually one or more of the following three areas are emphasized:
1. Education of patients and physicians regarding the specific area of concern to the organizaton.
2. Service programs designed to assist the patient to cope with his disease, to encourage early diagnosis and to refer patients to appropriate specialists and specialized care facilities.
3. Donation of funds for research into the cause, mechanism, prevention and cure of the disease relevant to each particular association.

ORGANIZATION

This varies from one agency to another but is usually composed of:
1. A board of directors or trustees consisting of physicians (minority) and lay (majority) representatives.
2. One or more Medical or Scientific Advisory Committees which formulate the general policies, plans and standards of the agency.
3. A large number of local affiliates which are primarily responsible for the delivery of services to patients at the local level.

In the section that follows we discuss the services available from these agencies. We strongly suggest that you contact the local affiliates in your area when you need assistance. We have listed the addresses of the national headquarters of each of these agencies for your information in case a local affiliate is not available.

NATIONAL COUNCIL ON ALCOHOLISM, INC.
2 Park Avenue
New York, NY 10016

General Information

This is the only national voluntary health agency founded to combat alcoholism. The council's major areas of activity are medical, labor-management, public information, education, research and evaluation, and community service programs. The National Council on Alcoholism and Alcoholics Anonymous are separate but they cooperate fully and supplement each other's work.

Specific Services Available to the Individual Patient

1. Alcoholism information centers.
2. Referral services for the alcoholic and families of alcoholics.
3. The distribution of more than one hundred different

special books and pamphlets of special interest to community leaders, families and individuals. A list of the currently available catalog of publications is published annually and is available on request from your local affiliate or from national headquarters.

ALLERGY FOUNDATON OF AMERICA
801 Second Avenue
New York, NY 10017

General Information

This agency was established to solve the health problems imposed by the allergic diseases.

Specific Services Available to the Individual Patient

1. Answers to specific questions about allergy.
2. Regional lists of allergists, clinics, hospitals and extended care facilities.
3. Educational pamphlets.

THE ARTHRITIS FOUNDATION
1212 Avenue of the Americas
New York, NY 10036

General Information

The Arthritis Foundation has stated its purposes as follows:

1. To increase local treatment facilities for arthritics.
2. To provide physicians more specialized education in the rheumatic diseases.
3. To increase the number of research scientists specializing in the rheumatic diseases.
4. To develop centers for research training and treatment.
5. To extend public knowledge of the human, social and economic costs of the rheumatic diseases and of what can be done to control and prevent them.
6. To raise, dispense and administer funds for these purposes.

Specific Services Available to the Individual Patient

1. Physical therapy in the home.
2. Handicrafts programs.
3. Funds for home care programs, visiting nurses, bed care, orthopedic appliances, self-help devices and drugs.
4. Educational pamphlets and leaflets.

THE NATIONAL FOUNDATION —
MARCH OF DIMES
Post Office Box 2000
White Plains, NY 10602

General Information

The mission of this organization is to organize and support research, education and service-oriented programs related to the causes, the means of prevention and the methods of treatment of birth defects.

Specific Services Available to the Individual Patient

1. A number of programs which encourage prenatal care by providing transportation, translation and baby-sitting for expectant mothers. Free clinics in many localities sponsor parent education and infant care classes.
2. Information concerning the use of german measles vaccine, Rh disease serum and genetic counseling.
3. Primary care at National Foundation–sponsored centers which are mainly concerned with the prenatal detection and prevention of birth defects.
4. Diagnosis and treatment of birth defects in children at National Foundation–sponsored medical service programs throughout the country.
5. Chapters occasionally provide financial assistance to patients with birth defects when no other resource is available.
6. A large number of pamphlets relating to the prevention, diagnosis and treatment of birth defects.

THE NATIONAL SOCIETY FOR THE
PREVENTION OF BLINDNESS, INC.
79 Madison Avenue
New York, NY 10016

General Information

The purposes of the society are to study and investigate any causes which may result in blindness or defective vision; to disseminate knowledge about all matters concerning the care, protection and use of the eyes; and to advocate measures which lead to the elimination of the causes of blindness.

Specific Services Available to the Individual Patient

1. Preschool vision screening programs available to children in inner cities and in migratory camps.
2. Glaucoma screening clinics for adults.
3. Home eye tests for preschoolers.
4. Referral to appropriate facilities or local eye care professionals in response to personal inquiries.
5. A variety of publications and films designed to educate the public about the major causes of eye injury and blindness.

FIGHT FOR SIGHT, INC.
41 W. 57th Street
New York, NY 10019

General Information

This organization is dedicated to the restoration and preservation of sight through eye research and treatment.

Specific Services Available to the Individual Patient

1. Referral to accredited clinics, eye physicians and agencies offering rehabilitation services.
2. Guidance to individuals requesting information concerning available sources for eye care.
3. Direct eye care at one of the four Fight for Sight children's eye clinics in New York City, Philadelphia, Pittsburgh and Newark, New Jersey.

THE NATIONAL ASSOCIATION FOR
VISUALLY HANDICAPPED
305 E. 24th Street
New York, NY 10010

General Information

This is the only national voluntary health agency devoted solely to the field of the partially seeing — not totally blind — individual.

Specific Services Available to the Individual Patient

1. A very wide variety of large-print publications ranging

from second grade to adult level reading materials, textbooks, novels and the like.
2. Information concerning services available for the partially sighted.
3. Rehabilitative, recreational, social and educational programs for partially sighted children and teenagers.
4. Counseling of the parents of partially sighted children.
5. Aid and assistance to the partially sighted, hospitalized veteran.
6. A catalog of large-type printed materials which can be purchased by partially sighted individuals or their families or schools can be obtained from the national headquarters.

THE AMERICAN FOUNDATION FOR THE BLIND
15 West 16th Street
New York, NY 10011

General Information

The general purpose of this foundation is to carry on research, to collect and disseminate information, and to advise and give counsel on matters that improve and strengthen services to blind persons.

Specific Services Available to the Individual Patient

1. Publication of books, magazines, monographs, and leaflets in ink print, large type, recorded and Braille forms.
2. Manufacture and sale of special aids and appliances for use by blind people; a seventy-two-page catalog is available upon request from the national headquarters.
3. Information, processing and distribution of identification cards for one-fare travel concessions for blind persons and a sighted companion. A pamphlet describing this service is available from the national headquarters.
4. An information and referral service which directs blind persons and their families to local agencies and institutions that can take care of their direct service needs.

THE AMERICAN CANCER SOCIETY
219 East 42nd Street
New York, NY 10017

General Information

The American Cancer Society is one of the largest and oldest voluntary health agencies in the United States. The society was founded to disseminate knowledge concerning the symptoms, treatment and prevention of cancer and to investigate conditions under which cancer is found.

Specific Services Available to the Individual Patient

1. Information and counseling, providing pertinent information and guidance through full use of community resources.
2. Loan and gift service which provides necessary and useful items for cancer patients such as surgical dressings, hospital beds, walkers, crutches, and gifts for the comfort and recreation of the patient such as lap robes and laryngectomy bibs.
3. Transportation service is provided as necessary for indigent cancer patients to and from approved treatment centers.
4. Depending on local needs and financial resources available, other services may be provided including medication, nursing and homemaker services and blood donor contacts.
5. A number of rehabilitation programs are available. These include programs for laryngectomy, mastectomy and ostomy patients. Psychological as well as physical rehabilitation is provided.
6. Cancer detection programs.
7. Tumor clinics for needy patients.
8. Limited, one-time, emergency financial aid.
9. A vast array of public education services are also provided by the society and are designed primarily to facilitate and encourage the early detection of cancer.

LEUKEMIA SOCIETY OF AMERICA, INC.
211 East 43rd Street
New York, NY 10017

General Information

The society is dedicated to the conquest of leukemia through medical research. In addition, the society supports patient aid and public and professional educational programs.

Specific Services Available to the Individual Patient

1. The society supports a program of supplementary financial assistance to patients with leukemia, the lymphomas, and Hodgkin's disease. It enables those who need it to obtain the lengthy and complex treatments required to control the serious disorders of the blood-forming organs. Information regarding this assistance program is available from national headquarters and from the local affiliates. In brief, assistance is available to qualified patients to cover payment for:
   a) drugs used in the care, treatment or control of leukemia and allied diseases
   b) transfusion of blood
   c) transportation to and from a doctor's office, hospital or treatment center
   d) x-ray therapy in amounts up to $300 for patients in the early stages of Hodgkin's disease when the disease is considered to be potentially curable.

2. A variety of educational literature and audiovisual material is available.

THE UNITED CEREBRAL PALSY ASSOCIATIONS, INC.
66 East 34th Street
New York, NY 10016

General Information

The purpose of this association is to promote diagnosis, treatment, education, rehabilitation and employment of persons with cerebral palsy and to encourage research.

Specific Services Available to the Individual Patient

1. A wide range of services and programs for individuals with cerebral palsy including:
   a) a program which concentrates on the motor and language development of preschoolers
   b) a youth activities program for handicapped teenagers including field trips, bowling, movies, dances and arts and crafts
   c) an adult development program which emphasizes the skills necessary for independent daily living, provides prevocational counseling, evaluation and training, individual instruction in specified subject areas and extensive creative and hobby type activities.

MEDICAL SERVICES AVAILABLE 131

2. Family counseling is offered as are parent education programs and conferences.
3. A cerebral palsy case registry and referral file is maintained as a service to families and other agencies serving the handicapped.
4. Preparation of handicapped persons for obtaining gainful employment.

THE NATIONAL CYSTIC FIBROSIS RESEARCH FOUNDATION
202 East 44th Street
New York, NY 10017

General Information

This organization operates for the benefit of scientific research, training and the dissemination of information with respect to cystic fibrosis and related diseases.

Specific Services Available to the Individual Patient

1. A wide variety of literature is available for the families of patients.
2. Local chapters are authorized to provide services to patients such as loans of equipment used in mist tent

therapy, transportation to clinics, low cost drug plans and the like.

THE AMERICAN DIABETES ASSOCIATION, INC.
18 East 48th Street
New York, NY 10017

General Information

The association has four major interests: patient education, professional education, public education and case finding, and research.

Specific Services Available to the Individual Patient

1. An annual diabetes detection drive.
2. Diabetes testing kits.
3. A variety of patient-oriented materials including a popular cookbook for diabetics, menu guides, carbohydrate exchange lists—this includes exchange lists for McDonald's, Chinese and Italian restaurants, and menus in several languages.
4. Regular education programs on diet, exercise, medication and complications of diabetes.
5. Physician referrals as well as city and county medical resources.
6. Summer camps for diabetic children.

THE EPILEPSY FOUNDATION OF AMERICA
733 15th Street, NW
Washington, DC 20005

General Information

The foundation sponsors research, education and service programs designed to make certain that people with epilepsy are properly integrated into all sectors of society.

Specific Services Available to the Individual Patient

A vast and comprehensive array of patient services are offered by the local chapters of this foundation. Space allows only a list of general categories of services available to patients. These include:

1. Counseling.
2. Information and referral services.
3. Educational services.
4. Financial assistance.
5. Transportation.
6. Employment and vocational rehabilitation.
7. Treatment.
8. Education and training.
9. Residential and day camps.
10. Special living arrangements.
11. Recreational programs.
12. Outpatient seizure clinics.
13. A wide variety of educational pamphlets, books and

leaflets designed to educate the patient and the family about the illness.

THE NATIONAL EASTER SEAL SOCIETY FOR CRIPPLED CHILDREN AND ADULTS
2023 West Ogden Avenue
Chicago, Illinois 60612

General Information

The primary purposes of this society are to provide rehabilitation services for the alleviation of physical, psychological, social and vocational effects of crippling diseases or injury; to conduct educational programs for the public, professional personnel, parents and families of crippled persons, and for employers, in order to create greater understanding of the crippled; and to support research.

Specific Services Available to the Individual Patient

A 211-page directory of services for the disabled is available from the national society. This is an exhaustive list of local chapters and the individual services which they offer in their areas. Space permits only a listing of the general services available through this organization which include:

1. Restorative services.
2. Information, referral and follow-up services.
3. Social and psychological services.
4. Equipment loan.
5. Recreation and camping.
6. Vocational services.
7. Educational services.
8. Transportation.

Furthermore, a vast library of publications as well as books and films are available to patients at a nominal cost.

THE AMERICAN HEART ASSOCIATION, INC.
44 East 23rd Street
New York, NY 10010

General Information

The primary purpose of this agency is to support research, professional and public education and community services with the objective of reducing death and disability from the cardiovascular diseases.

Specific Services Available to the Individual Patient

1. Consumer education through nationwide radio and television public service announcements, films, posters, volunteer speakers and magazine articles.
2. Programs to help people change their eating habits, i.e., food fairs, diet and weight control programs, nutritional counseling to schools, restaurants and hospitals.
3. Screening programs for high blood pressure.
4. Rehabilitation for heart attack and stroke patients and retraining their families.
5. Implementation of programs in cardiopulmonary resuscitation through manuals and films.
6. A vast array of literature available to the individual concerning smoking, diet, cholesterol, heart murmurs, blood pressure, exercise, specific medications, congenital heart diseases, pacemakers, coronary care units, strokes and other cardiovascular-related topics.
7. Diet charts and menu planning aids for patients on fat-controlled or sodium restricted diets.

THE NATIONAL HEMOPHILIA FOUNDATION
25 West 39th Street
New York, NY 10018

General Information

The foundation is dedicated to the support of basic research and clinical study of hemophilia and related coagulation disorders, to disseminating knowledge relating to these diseases, and to organizing chapters in order to develop and expand treatment and services for the care of the hemophiliac.

Specific Services Available to the Individual Patient

The foundation sponsors and fosters a number of services available to the patient such as:

1. Development of comprehensive care clinics which can fill the need for both good medical care and supportive psychological and social services.
2. The encouragement of summer camp programs for hemophilic children.
3. The encouragement of the United Air Lines Pilot Association program which provides free airlifts of hemophilic children to treatment centers where they can receive therapy not available in their hometowns.
4. Help with the cost of hospital care in indigent cases.
5. Aid for rehabilitation in cases of hemophilic joint disease.
6. Supplies of blood and plasma.
7. Financial support to clinics and treatment centers. A directory of hemophilia treatment centers is available from national headquarters.

THE NATIONAL COUNCIL FOR HOMEMAKER-HOME HEALTH AIDE SERVICES, INC.
1740 Broadway
New York, NY 10019

General Information

The council's purpose is to stimulate expansion and improvement of homemaker-home health aide services throughout the country.

Specific Services Available to the Individual Patient

Homemaker-home health aides provide service in the areas of:

1. Child care.
2. Maintenance of the home.
3. Problems of the aging and personal care.
4. A national directory of services is available from the general headquarters.

Contact your local affiliate for further information regarding the local availability of these services in your area.

THE NATIONAL KIDNEY FOUNDATION, INC.
315 Park Avenue South
New York, NY 10010

General Information

The objective of this foundation is to improve the care, treatment and prevention of kidney diseases both in the hospital and the community.

Specific Services Available to the Individual Patient

1. Information and referral for persons needing medical care.
2. Information on available financial resources for persons with kidney diseases.
3. Detection program: a bacteriuria testing program for urinary tract infections in girls is carried out in selected elementary schools.
4. Blood bank: the foundation maintains an account with the Red Cross so that blood is available to kidney patients who need it.
5. Drug bank: drugs are made available at cost to kidney patients whose doctors are members of the Foundation.
6. Medic Alert emblems: emblems which identify the wearer as a dialysis or kidney transplant patient are made available free of charge to those patients who can't afford them.
7. Education: the affiliates provide information services which assist those afflicted with a kidney disease to make use of all resources available in their communities.
8. The local affiliates are also involved in the recruitment of donors for kidney transplants.

PLANNED PARENTHOOD – WORLD
POPULATION
810 7th Avenue
New York, NY 10019

General Information

The major objective of this organization is to provide leadership in making effective means of voluntary fertility control available and accessible to all.

Specific Services Available to the Individual Patient

Local affiliates provide a variety of services such as:

1. The operation of licensed medical facilities and centers which provide a full range of medical and counseling services related to:
   a) fertility
   b) prescription and nonprescription contraception methods
   c) pregnancy detection
   d) early abortion
   e) voluntary sterilization
   f) infertility
   g) gonorrhea testing and treatment
   h) breast and cervical cancer detection
   i) adoption referral
   j) sex education

   Such centers are staffed by gynecologists, social

workers and registered nurses, nurse midwives, nurse clinicians and volunteers and are open usually on Saturdays and evenings as well as regular daytime hours.

NATIONAL MULTIPLE SCLEROSIS SOCIETY
257 Park Avenue South
New York, NY 10010

General Information

The society is dedicated to discovering the cause, treatment and cure for multiple sclerosis. As the cause of this disease remains unknown, the society's major concern is in research, although patient services are provided through the local chapters.

Specific Services Available to the Individual Patient

1. Guidance and counseling on physical, emotional, social and economic problems to patients and families by a Medical Advisory Committee.
2. Distribution of such items as wheelchairs, hospital beds, walkers and clothing.
3. Referrals and transportation to medical facilities.
4. Recreation programs for home-bound and ambulatory patients.

5. Occupational and physical therapy and Visiting Nurse and homemaker services are often made available through grants by local chapters to community agencies.
6. Direct medical care provided by a variety of multiple sclerosis clinics, rehabilitation clinics, university-associated clinics and community hospital neurological clinics which are supported in part by funds contributed by local chapters.

THE MUSCULAR DYSTROPHY ASSOCIATIONS OF AMERICA, INC.
1790 Broadway
New York, NY 10019

General Information

The objectives of the associations are to foster scientific research into the cause and cure of muscular dystrophy and related neuromuscular diseases and to render services to patients with these diseases.

Specific Services Available to the Individual Patient

1. Financial assistance in the purchase and repair of a variety of orthopedic appliances such as walkers and crutches, braces, orthopedic shoes, night splints, wheelchairs and accessories, surgical corsets, hospital beds and the like.

2. Financial assistance for medically prescribed physical therapy on a limited basis.
3. Transportation for clinic visits, dental appointments, chapter-sponsored recreational activities, attendance at school, to and from employment.
4. Recreational programs.
5. Financial assistance to pay for influenza inoculations recommended by physicians.
6. Extensive and comprehensive financial assistance for medical care when provided by one of the many outpatient clinics which have been established by the Muscular Dystrophy Associations of America. These services include:
    a) complete diagnostic examinations including laboratory tests and even short-term hospitalization if necessary
    b) physical therapy under medical supervision
    c) assistance by the clinic's medical social worker with personal and family problems
    d) genetic counseling
    e) occupational therapy
    f) quarterly medical evaluations
    g) follow-up clinic visits

THE MYASTHENIA GRAVIS
FOUNDATION, INC.
2 East 103rd Street
New York, NY 10029

General Information

The major aims and purposes of the foundation are to foster and support research into the cause, prevention, alleviation and cure of myasthenia gravis and to voluntarily aid and assist the sufferers of this disease.

Specific Services Available to the Individual Patient

1. Drug banks which supply medications on physicians' prescriptions.
2. Information and referral services.
3. A network of free or low-cost clinics devoted to patient care is sponsored by the organization.

THE NATIONAL PARAPLEGIA FOUNDATION
333 North Michigan Avenue
Chicago, Illinois 60601

General Information

The major purposes of the foundation are to foster and promote spinal cord injury research and to advocate adequate care for paraplegics.

Specific Services Available to the Individual Patient

1. Information and referral to appropriate physicians and clinics for care.
2. Equipment loan and repair.
3. Transportation for medical services.
4. Assistance in finding gainful employment.
5. Referral to sources of financial assistance.
6. A vast array of literature designed to teach the paraplegic how to care for himself, maintain his health, regain a certain degree of mobility, and readjust to society.

The foregoing is only a partial list of the total number of National Voluntary Health Agencies in the United States. We have focused our attention on those agencies which provide specific services to individual patients. There are numerous other voluntary associations which are equally as praiseworthy as the ones mentioned but they were not listed in this chapter because they are primarily involved in the support of research, professional education, political awareness, or were limited in scope to one or two very restricted localities.

8

What You Need to Know before Choosing a Nursing Home

Contributed by Lorena Thorup, B.S.,R.N.

THE SPECIAL COMMITTEE ON AGING of the United States Senate has recently issued a report stating that "long-term care for older Americans stands today as the most troubled and troublesome component of our entire health care system." The magnitude of the problem is illustrated by the following statistics: in 1900, the average life span in the United States was forty-seven years; today it is seventy years. Since chronic, debilitating disease frequently strikes this group of elderly citizens they commonly require continuing and extended nursing care. Ironically, as longevity has increased in our society, so has job mobility. Consequently the family that formerly would have taken care of its ailing and elderly members may now be widely dispersed and dependent on the services of a nursing home or other type of extended care facility.

Since most of the elderly population live on small fixed incomes, the nursing home industry that has developed to fill this need has had to face the problem of providing high quality care at a low, affordable cost.

Many individual nursing homes have met this challenge and capably provide skilled and compassionate care at acceptable rates. There are many others, however, which have made their owners wealthy by providing the least expensive and most inadequate services at the highest possible cost.

Such unethical practices have been possible because federal and state guidelines, which must be met before a home can qualify for Medicare or Medicaid payments, have been in a continuous state of flux. The confusion which naturally accompanies these conditions creates the opportunity for unscrupulous parties to defraud the public. Furthermore, state and federal inspectors who periodically visit each nursing home to ensure compliance with current guidelines frequently perform inadequate inspections either because they are insufficiently trained for their jobs or because they themselves are confused by the guidelines.

The care of elderly patients can only be provided by sufficient numbers of skilled personnel trained to recognize and understand the problems peculiar to this age group. However, the 1974 Senate report "Nursing Home Care in the United States: Failure in Public Policy" states that 80–90 percent of nursing home personnel are untrained nurses' aides and orderlies, "most literally hired off the streets." It goes on to say that in 1971 "there were 5.3 nursing home employees for every 10 nursing home patients and that by contrast general and surgical hospitals averaged 26 employees for every 10 patients."

Until the day arrives when all nursing homes are supervised, inspected and accredited by responsible agencies similar to the Joint Commission on Accreditation of Hospitals (JCAH), when all bedside nursing personnel are required to be trained and licensed, when inspectors learn to enforce appropriate regulations and when ample numbers of registered and licensed nurses are required to staff these facilities, there is no alternative but to provide consumers with information necessary to evaluate each nursing home for themselves. Certain nursing homes are currently accredited by the JCAH. The majority of these are administered and staffed by JCAH-accredited hospitals although some are independent institutions. A list of these can be found in a publication of The American Hospital Association entitled *The AHA Guide to the Health Care Field*, which should be available in your public library.

There are various types of nursing homes which can be classified according to the type of care they provide.

"Skilled Nursing Care" refers to a facility which is required to provide twenty-four-hour nursing supervision by a Registered or a Licensed Vocational or Licensed Practical Nurse, plus many constantly changing detailed requirements related to facilities and direct patient care.

"Intermediate Care" refers to a facility which is required to provide only part-time licensed nursing supervision each week and which serves patients all of whom are ambulatory.

"Mental Hygiene Care" refers to a facility which provides a security environment to patients with mental or marked behavior problems.

These three classifications of homes are required to be licensed and inspected by the agency so designated in each state.

Homes operating under these classifications are likewise approved to receive payments from the Medicaid program for those patients who are unable to meet all or a portion of the costs. Medicaid is a welfare program financed jointly by state and federal governments.

Only homes operating under the "Skilled Nursing" category may be approved to receive funds from Medicare; however, increasingly strict eligibility requirements have resulted in few and only short term reimbursements from the program at this writing.

There are many excellent nursing homes with dedicated owners, administrators and nurses who choose to operate quality institutions. May this chapter help you to find them.

Before You Look

Your physician will probably recommend one of the locally available nursing homes according to your particular needs as well as other considerations such as its location and cost. Before you accept his recommendation ask the following questions:

1. Is the Physician Willing to Visit Any Nursing Home You Choose?

If the home you select is far from your physician's office he may be unable to visit regularly. You should be prepared to either select another home or arrange to be referred to a nearby physician.

2. Is the Home Acceptable to Your Personal Insurance Company or to Governmental Assistance Programs?

Most insurance companies pay only reliable licensed homes. If you cannot fully finance the costs of care and therefore need financial assistance, you should contact a nursing home administrator or a social worker for information and referral to such sources as Medicare (national), Supplementary Security Income (national), Medicaid (state and national), Champus (military) and Veterans Administration (postmilitary).

3. Is the Location Convenient for Frequent Visiting, Particularly If You Do Not Drive?

Regular visits by friends and relatives are essential for the well-being of nursing home residents who need familiar human contact for their well-being and peace of mind.

4. Is the Location Relatively Free of Traffic and Airplane Noise?

A tranquil environment permits patients to obtain the rest and sleep necessary to maintain their health and to recuperate from many illnesses.

When you are looking for a nursing home, you should plan for sufficient time to interview the administrator, talk to the staff, and look around for yourself. You should be welcomed to do so.

Ready to Look: What to Look For

THE BUILDING

1. Is the Building Constructed So That No More than Thirty-five Patients Are Assigned to Each Nursing Station?

It is very difficult for a team of nurses, orderlies and aides to provide adequate care for more than 30–35 patients. This is especially true if some or all of the patients are bedfast and unable to get about without assistance.

2. Are the Kitchen Facilities Large Enough and Arranged for Efficient Handling of Food?

If a kitchen is crowded, if refrigerators are not ample, if open sink dishwashing facilities are near to food and if cupboards are cluttered and messy, the preparation of food may not be sanitary or safe.

3. Are Bathroom Facilities Available between Each Two Rooms or for Each Room?

Whether or not the patient is able to walk there should be a bathroom available between each two rooms. A bathtub or shower is not particularly important as patients may be bathed in a separate facility where lifts or shower chairs facilitate safe bathing and shampooing. A toilet and lavatory are essential not only for ambulatory patients but also to permit prompt emptying of bedpans, urinals and mouth care basins and rinsing of soiled bed linen.

All bathrooms should have high toilets equipped with grab bars for the comfort and safety of the patients. Equipment for flushing and cleansing bedpans should be provided and plenty of towels, washcloths and soap should be present.

4. Is the Building Large Enough So That Patients Can Be Placed in Different Groups (Such as Bedfast,

CHOOSING A NURSING HOME

Wheelchair or Ambulatory) to Facilitate Economy in Staff Assignments as Well as in Fees Charged?

Some large homes adjust their fees according to the amount of care each patient will require. Obviously a patient who is able to walk, dress and eat without assistance doesn't need as much nursing care or linen as a helpless bedfast patient requires.

5. Is the Building Heated by Controlled Central Heat?

Controlled central heat assures safety as well as uniformity of temperature and avoidance of drafts.

6. Does the Building Have Air Conditioning for Hot Summer Days?

7. Is the Bedside Bell System Functioning Well and Is It Easily Accessible to the Patient?

The call system is extremely important because it may be the only means of calling for help. This is especially important during evening and night hours when there are fewer employees per patient than during the day.

8. Is There an Outdoor Area Equipped with Chairs, Tables and Shade?

An outdoor patio area serves as a welcome change from

the patient's room and also provides a quiet semiprivate retreat for visitors.

9. Is There a Recreation Room for Social Activities?

Many patients are active enough to use a recreation room, especially if it is adequately equipped with games and craft materials. Less active patients enjoy watching the others. In either case, the opportunity for socialization is invaluable.

PERSONNEL

Eighty to ninety percent of the bedside care in nursing homes today is provided by nurses' aides and orderlies who are not required to be either licensed or trained to care for the elderly. This astonishing situation is currently under investigation by two U.S. Senate subcommittees and has attracted the attention of several concerned professional organizations as well as the press. Little progress has been made to rectify this condition as of this writing. Until adequate legislative measures are taken which make such training mandatory, the wise consumer should carefully examine the quality and quantity of the personnel at several nursing homes before he selects one for himself or a loved one.

CHOOSING A NURSING HOME 155

WHAT YOU NEED TO KNOW ABOUT PERSONNEL

1. **Is the Administrator Knowledgeable and Seemingly Compassionate? Is the Administrator a Member of the Local "Nursing Home Association" or Equivalent Professional Group?**

2. **How Many Licensed Nurses Are Employed? Licensed Nurses Are Either Registered Nurses or Vocational Nurses.**

Registered Nurses are known throughout the United States as RN's. Their education may have been a two to three year course in vocational schools, or a four to five year course in a college or university.

Vocational or Licensed Practical Nurses are educated in private or vocational trade schools. Their education usually requires one year, which leads to a Certificate or Diploma and licensure.

Both Registered Nurses, Vocational Nurses and Licensed Practical Nurses must pass examinations and secure state licensure before they can legally practice nursing.

Currently 20 percent or less of the bedside nursing staff in nursing homes are Licensed Nurses. This figure should be much higher to provide optimal care. Spend the time necessary to find the nursing home in your community with the highest percentage of Licensed Nurses on its staff.

3. How Many Nurses' Aides or Orderlies Are Employed?

Nurses' aides and orderlies comprise a national average of 80 percent to 90 percent of the bedside care staff. As we have already mentioned, they are not required to be trained or licensed at this time.

Nurses' aides and orderlies provide much of the actual bedside care of the patients. This consists of bathing; mouth, hair and nail care; linen changing; bedmaking; attention to toileting; assistance with walking and wheelchairs; frequent turning if the patient is bedfast; feeding; irrigating of catheters; care of flowers, clothing, bedside tables and wheelchairs; and other duties intended to provide comfort.

Whereas little training is necessary to prepare a nurses' aide or orderly to perform these functions, in many nursing homes with low numbers of Licensed Nurses the untrained personnel are often assigned many skilled nursing duties for which they are not prepared.

We do not intend to deny the importance of the nurses' aide or orderly. They are necessary for the operation of the nursing home and provide an important personal service to the patients. The basic problem is that since their wages are lower than what Licensed Nurses are paid the nursing home owner often tries to cut costs by hiring fewer trained and licensed personnel than he actually needs. Skilled nursing duties then naturally must be delegated to unskilled personnel.

4. Does the Nurse in Charge Make Out Daily Patient Care and Need Assignment Schedules for Each Aide or Orderly on Duty?

Since staff and patient location changes from day to day, it is essential that each aide be given an assignment in writing. There should also be posted a list of clearly defined duties and limitations for all untrained bedside personnel.

5. Are Physicians' Visits Accompanied by the Nurse in Charge?

Both the nurse and the physician are better able to assess the progress and the problems of the patient in this fashion.

6. Does the Director of the Nursing Staff Provide for Periodic In-Service Training for all Nursing Personnel?

Regardless of ample staff and qualified personnel, frequent in-service instruction is essential.

7. Is There an Employee Whose Duty It Is to Clean and Supply Rooms and Bathroom Facilities Daily?

There should be daily service to assure sufficient supplies of linen, soap and toilet paper.

8. Are Barbers and Beauticians Available?

A room specially equipped for the use of barbers and beauticians is a valuable asset to patients who are ambulatory, as well as to many who may be brought in on stretchers. The majority of homes provide such facilities. Patients are expected to pay the employees who come in from their shops to serve them.

9. Does the Staff Appear to Be Kind, Thoughtful and Interested in Patients' Welfare?

When looking around, one can usually judge whether the staff appears to be truly interested in their work and in the welfare and contentment of the patients.

CARE OF PATIENTS

1. How Often Are Baths Scheduled?

Baths should be scheduled at least twice a week or more often if indicated by illness or inability to keep clean.

2. How Often Is Linen Changed?

Linen should be changed routinely at least once a week or as often as needed to keep the patients clean and the room free of odors.

3. Is Attention Given to Trimming Nails?

Finger and toenails should be trimmed and filed as a feature of the bath. Neglected and painful problems should be referred to a podiatrist, whose fee is not usually included in the weekly price for care.

4. Does There Appear to Be Sufficient Staff to Avoid Offensive Odors, Neglected Care and Messy Rooms?

Odors and clutter cannot be avoided at all times but should be removed as quickly as possible on all shifts. Incontinent patients should be checked routinely at frequent intervals.

5. Do Aides and Orderlies Have Time to Help Patients Who Need Assistance with Walking?

Many long-term patients lose the ability or the desire to walk unless they are given daily encouragement and assistance. This form of exercise is essential to prevent bedsores, improve circulation, maintain muscle tone, and enhance self-esteem.

6. Are the Patients Who Are Unable to Feed Themselves Fed Carefully and Slowly?

Some homes charge an additional fee when a patient needs help with feeding. Often part-time employees, or semi-volunteers come in for this purpose. If these patients are grouped together, one aide or volunteer can feed two at the same time, thus defraying some of the cost.

7. Is Ample Time Scheduled to Allow the Patients Who Can Feed Themselves to Eat Slowly?

The long-term-care patient tends to eat slowly since all movements are inclined to be slow. The home should provide meals in a pleasant, spacious dining room for ambulatory as well as wheelchair patients. The only social contact that many patients have is at mealtime. Such arrangements are, therefore, of inestimable value.

8. Are there Facilities or Arrangements for Rehabilitation as Ordered by the Patient's Physician, such as Massage, Muscle Training, Speech Therapy and Relearning to Walk?

Only large homes are apt to provide facilities for daily rehabilitation therapy and if so, such homes are usually combined with a hospital.

Some homes offer rehabilitation therapy by bringing in therapists as indicated by physicians' orders. Many patients respond to rehabilitation training and therapy miraculously and are therefore often able to return to their homes with the assistance of volunteers, family or professional homemaker services.

9. Are Medicines Crushed and Administered in Juice or Sauce for Patients Who Have Difficulty in Swallowing?

Some infirm patients are unable to swallow solid capsule medications. They may place such capsules or pills in their mouths then expectorate them when the nurse has moved away. A careful nurse will label medicine tickets to state "crush" if indicated. The crushed medications are then placed in juice or a sweetened sauce which enables the patient to swallow easily and eliminates bitter tastes.

10. Are Patients' Teeth Cared for by the Patient or the Aide at Least during Morning Care?

Mouth and teeth care should be a routine duty whether the patient is bedfast or ambulatory.

11. Are Linen Shelves Supplied with Ample Linen to Assure That All Patients Are Continuously Clean and Dry?

A glance at the linen cupboards will reveal much information about the nursing care. A linen cupboard frequently empty obviously implies that patients cannot at all times be clean, dry and free of odors.

12. Does the Home Provide for Patients' Personal Laundry? If So, Is There an Additional Fee?

The majority of homes provide for personal laundry on the premises. Some charge an additional fee for the service. A common problem is lost clothing, due largely to fading name labels or to clothing being placed in another patient's room. If all personal clothing is well labeled upon admittance and if a specified employee is assigned to this task, such losses and confusion can be avoided.

13. Are There Ample Wheelchairs, Walkers, Canes or Crutches for Those Who Need Such Aids, or Are You Required to Provide Them?

Some homes supply such equipment; however, it is advisable to inquire about additional fees which may be charged. Purchasing your own equipment may be more economical. If so, make arrangements for obvious name plates which cannot be easily lost or become faded.

14. Are Money and Valuables such as Watches, Rings, and Possibly Razors, Labeled and Locked in the Nursing Station to Assure Their Safety?

FACILITIES IN ROOMS

1. Is Each Room Equipped So That Each Patient has a Bedside Table with Sufficient Drawer Space for Personal Needs?

2. Is There Sufficient Closet Space to Hang Clothing and to Store Shoes and Slippers off the Floor?

Since a nursing home is now the patient's home, there are needs, physical as well as psychological, for considerably more clothing, artifacts, books, etc., than are required when in a short term facility or a hospital.

3. Is There Space in the Closet for Blankets, Luggage and Other Bulky Personal Objects?

If such items must be stored on the floor, it is difficult to keep the closet clean and free of insects.

4. Is There Also a Table for Photographs, Flowers, Craft Work and Other Personal Needs?

Such a table is a very essential asset for the happiness of a patient who is mentally able to enjoy activities and memories.

5. Are the Bedside Tables and the Closets Kept Free from Clutter?

6. Is There at Least One Comfortable Chair per Person in Each Room?

Some patients prefer to remain in their rooms at all times. Chairs are also essential for visiting in privacy either with other patients or with family and friends.

7. Are Patients Permitted to Decorate Their Own Rooms?

SANITATION

1. Are Bedside Water Containers Cleansed and Sterilized Periodically?

2. Is Dishwashing Adequate?

Ask if the home uses a dishwasher which ensures a high enough temperature to destroy disease-causing organisms.

3. Are There Facilities for Periodic Sterilizing of Bedpans and Urinals?

There are sterilizers made specifically for bedpans and

urinals. If large numbers of these items must be sterilized a regular autoclave may be used.

4. Is Garbage Removed Frequently?

5. Does the Home Appear to Be Clean and Well Organized?

SAFETY

1. Are There Enough Exits, Clearly Marked, and Are All of the Exit Doors Locked Only from the Outside?

In the event of fire or other disaster it is essential that patients be able to leave the building at all times. Room doors should seldom be locked but if absolutely necessary, they should be locked only from the outside to permit escape.

2. Are Sprinklers or Fire Extinguishers in Evidence?

New buildings are usually equipped with sprinklers. Many buildings, however, rely on fire extinguishers, which need to be checked periodically. Directions for operating fire extinguishers should be clearly printed within easy view. There should be periodic demonstrations and fire drills for the entire staff.

3. Are Grab Bars Installed Next to Each Toilet, in Bath and Shower Rooms, and in All Hallways to Facilitate Walking and Changing Position?

Grab bars are either metal or wood rails firmly attached to walls at about hand height.

4. Are All Floors Free of Slippery Wax?

Many homes are carpeted, particularly in hallways and recreation areas. If not, a non-slippery wax should be used.

5. Are Hallways Wide Enough to Permit Ease of Passing for Walkers and Wheelchairs?

If hallways are not wide enough for this purpose, the fire department and the inspector should be notified.

6. Are Steps Absent from Areas That Patients Use Every Day?

Steps are very hazardous and should not be in areas occupied by patients.

7. Are There Rules Restricting Smoking Except in Designated Areas?

Smoking in rooms is too dangerous to be permitted.

Smoke is also offensive to many patients; therefore, there should be a designated area, easily observable to the staff, set aside for smokers.

RECREATION

1. Are Arrangements Made for Activities such as Games, Cards, Music and Crafts for Those Who Choose and Are Able to Participate?

Many homes arrange for recreational activities within the needs and the life-style of the patients. Some long-term care patients are no longer interested in social activities. If so they should not be pushed to participate.

2. Are Books and Magazines Available for Those Interested in Reading?

Books, newspapers and magazines should be available for the patients who are interested in reading.

3. Are There Volunteers Who Provide Personal Attention such as Letter Writing and Shopping?

Volunteers contribute greatly to the happiness of patients in nursing homes. Many patients have no relatives or close friends to visit them or to attend to their personal needs.

4. Is Visiting Encouraged and Are Visiting Hours Flexible?

The majority of homes encourage visiting in the afternoon and evening. Visiting in the morning is not encouraged because of interference with patient care. Closely restricted visiting hours could be a reason for looking elsewhere.

5. Are Arrangements Made for Sunday Religious Services?

Many patients are eager to participate in religious services regardless of the denomination. With advancing age, religion becomes more meaningful and necessary for many. Many churches are happy to provide short services and music on a scheduled basis.

FOOD

1. Is the Food Well Prepared, Appetizing and Attractive?

It is advisable to visit a home at mealtime so that you can

observe the quality of the food and look at the weekly menus.

2. Are Menu Plans and Food Preparation Approved by a Licensed Dietician?

Well-qualified and licensed dieticians usually supervise food services in nursing homes. They are concerned with food preparation, sanitation and safety as well as with menu planning to assure palatable, nutritious and easily chewed food.

3. Are Menus Also Planned to Comply with Physicians' Orders and Patients' Needs for Special Diets such as Diabetic, Low Residue and Low Sodium?

A licensed dietician is qualified to plan all special diets as ordered by physicians. In her absence the supervising nurse is often called upon to plan menus.

4. Does the Kitchen Equipment Appear to Be Adequate?

Delivery carts should be accurately labeled with each patient's name and room number so that patients on special diets may be assured of receiving the correct tray.

5. Are There Ample Refrigerators for Food Storage?

There should be sufficient refrigerators to store all perishable food and frozen foods. Leftover food should never be left on stoves or counters for any length of time because of the danger of bacterial contamination and food poisoning.

Costs of a Nursing Home

Costs in a nursing home vary somewhat with the category and ownership of the home as well as with the thoroughness of services offered. Most homes are operated as business investments planned for profit.

It is important that you understand what is included in the weekly price. It would be to your advantage to ask for a written statement of the following services:

1. Is Personal Laundry Included?

If not, ask about the fee and how arrangements are made for this service.

2. Are Any Medicines Ordered by Your Physician Included?

If not, do you have the privilege of securing prescription medicines at your choice of a pharmacy? If you live in an area where pharmacy prices vary greatly, you should be given this privilege.

3. Are Treatment, First Aid Materials or Personal Supplies Included?

There may be an additional charge for items such as Band-Aids, bandages, ointments, catheters, enemas, suppositories, cathartics, toothpaste and Kleenex.

4. Is There an Extra Charge for Wheelchairs, Walkers, and Other Mechanical Devices Used to Assist with Ambulation?

In general, the cost of nursing home care can vary greatly depending upon a large number of variables such as:

Location
Type of building
Quality and quantity of employees
Menu
Supporting services
Profit margin
Efficiency of administration

Many well-managed and well-staffed homes provide adequate and even excellent services at average fees. Many poorly managed and inadequately staffed homes which offer unimportant frills may charge unrealistically high prices.

If the consumer is aware that assistance is available from private and military insurance companies as well as from Medicaid, he should be able to obtain adequate care for the patient in need in an average or minimum cost nursing home.

What You Can Do to Help the Nursing Home and the Patient

1. You could visit often; even though you may not appear to be recognized, perhaps you really are.
2. If you visit at mealtime, you could offer to feed the patient if assistance is needed.
3. You could help immensely by labeling all of the patient's clothing with wash-proof name labels.
4. You could make a nylon mesh zippered laundry bag in which all of the patient's clothing could be laundered and dried. Such a bag can save much time otherwise spent sorting the clothing and helps assure safe return of all items.
5. You could attend to mending, replacing buttons and removing worn clothing.
6. You could clean the bedside table of clutter and provide an ample supply of personal needs such as comb, brush, toothbrush, mirror, etc.
7. If approved by the physician, you could assist the patient with walking if necessary.
8. You could take care of fresh flowers and plants.
9. You could plan periodic short trips away from the nursing home, to your home or to other recreational facilities, if the patient is able to go.

It is your privilege to be firm in expecting adequate care, but keep in mind that nursing in a nursing home is hard work for all of the staff. Every move of most patients is on a much slower scale than when they were able-bodied. Eating, moving about, thinking, taking medicines, in fact all actions, are much more time-consuming than is readily recognized.

Many nursing home administrators would like to employ a larger staff with a higher number of licensed nurses but they are faced with problems of rising costs and pressures from owners. As you look about, however, you will probably note that the most efficient, well-organized and pleasant homes also have ample and well-selected employees to provide for the needs of the patients.

9

The Consumer and the Cost of Preserving His Health

1. Generic versus Brand Name Drugs: Cost versus Quality
2. Anticipating the Cost of Your Medical Care
3. Essentials of an Adequate Health Insurance Plan

1. GENERIC VERSUS BRAND NAME DRUGS: COST VERSUS QUALITY

When you select a physician you are making a choice that affects not only the quality of medical care you will receive but also how much it will cost. In addition to your doctor's professional fee you will also assume a number of other expenses the size of which is determined in large part by decisions which the doctor makes on your behalf. The most obvious of these additional expenses are laboratory fees, consultant fees, and the cost of prescription drugs. There is not much you can do to lessen the laboratory or consultant fees. In contrast, there is a great deal you can do to lower your drug bill.

Nearly six billion dollars is spent annually by the American public for prescription drugs (see Reference number 1 at end of this section). The average cost for every man, woman and child, therefore, amounts to $30 per year, or $120 annually for a family of four. Actually these costs are not distributed evenly throughout society but are borne most heavily by the aged and by families with young children, who generally require more medical attention than the rest of us. The annual cost for prescription drugs can easily amount to several hundred dollars to these individuals, and they are usually least able to afford it. It is obvious that some relief from these expenditures is necessary. Recently, much attention has been given to this matter by several professional and consumer-oriented publications (see References 2 to 4) which have dealt with the relative cost of "brand name" versus "generic" drugs.

"Brand name" drugs are those which are manufactured by large pharmaceutical companies and sold under a particular trade name. For example, Omnipen, Penbriten, Principen/N, Pen A/N, Supen and Amcill are some of the brand names for ampicillin (the generic name for this drug). Pharmaceutical companies spend a great deal of money advertising their products to physicians who, like everybody else, are susceptible to the influence of well-designed promotional campaigns. Since nearly 90 percent of all prescriptions are for brand name drugs (see Reference 1), the effectiveness of this advertising is obvious. The term "generic" when applied to a drug refers to its chemical name or to simplified versions of that name. There are many, usually smaller, pharmaceutical companies which manufacture these drugs and sell them to pharmacies without labeling them with a particular brand name. Hence, these drugs are referred to as "generics." The wholesale cost of "generics" may be substantially lower than equivalent "brand name" drugs for a number of reasons, not the least of which is the difference in advertising costs.

If the quality of a given "generic" drug can be shown to be equivalent to its "brand name" counterpart (see below), the consumer could realize a substantial savings in drug costs by "buying generic." Given the realities of current prescribing practices, however, it will take a certain degree of effort for you to actually reap these benefits. First of all, your physician may not realize that there are "generics" available as substitutes for a particular "brand name" drug he commonly prescribes. Secondly, he may be reluctant to switch from the "brand name" drug with which he is familiar to the relatively unknown "generic" for a variety of reasons, most importantly his uncertainty as to the quality of the "generic" drug (see below). Third, even if the physician does prescribe a "generic" drug the pharmacist is not obliged to dispense it unless the physician insists upon it. Fourth, the pharmacist doesn't always pass on the savings of the lower wholesale cost of generic drugs to the patient.

The first three of these obstacles can be dealt with by

a frank discussion with your doctor concerning the reason for his selection of a particular product when he writes out a prescription for you. *Do not be embarrassed or too timid to ask; it is your money he is spending and your health which is at stake.* The adequacy, and courtesy, of his response to these questions will give you some insight into the adequacy of his knowledge and willingness to learn. Certainly no one physician can, or should, be an expert on the relative merits of all "brand name" versus "generic" drugs, but every doctor should know about the drugs he commonly prescribes and he should be willing to try to find out what is known about any particular drug you inquire about.

The last of the four obstacles we mentioned above, namely the fact that pharmacists don't always pass the savings on "generic" drugs along to the consumer, can be solved by comparison shopping. This is especially true when you are going to be taking a particular drug for a long time, because the savings can be substantial. Prices vary widely from pharmacy to pharmacy and in some cases the price of a drug in one pharmacy may be one-half to one-third of the price at another. In a recent study of thirty-three pharmacies in a large city in upstate New York it was found that "generic prescribing was no guarantee of savings. Brand name drugs at chain pharmacies often cost less than generic products in independent stores, and in a few cases generic prescriptions were filled at a higher price than brand name prescriptions in the same pharmacy. Prices and savings varied widely from one pharmacy to another. . . ." (Reference 5). The authors concluded that "clearly, it can pay to shop around."

The all important question, of course, which arises in any discussion of "brand name" versus "generic" drugs deals with the problem of determining the quality of the individual product. "Quality," in terms of prescription and nonprescription drugs, is a general term which refers to the product's efficacy and safety as well as to the uniformity of drug content from tablet to tablet and the stability of the drug over a period of time. No general statement concerning the relative quality of "generic" as opposed to "brand name" drugs can be made at the present time. Indeed, the Office of Technology Assessment of the U.S. Congress has recently reported that current regulatory practices of federal watchdog agencies do not assure "bioequivalence for drug products" (Reference 6). "Bioequivalence" is medical jargon that refers to the ability of the body to extract the same amount of active drug from one pill as from another and from one manufacturer to another, and obviously is a very important factor in determining the efficacy and safety of any particular product.

Although the Food and Drug Administration and many academic and pharmaceutical research laboratories are currently working on the problem it will be many years until valid scientific information concerning the relative "quality" of similar drug products will be available for the majority of commonly prescribed medicines. For the present, the consumer must therefore depend on his doctor's judgment in each individual case.

In summary, based on the above discussion you should be aware of the following:

1. Just because a drug falls into the "generic" category doesn't mean it is inferior to its "brand name" equivalent . . . nor does it mean it is superior.
2. The price of drugs in both categories varies widely from pharmacy to pharmacy but usually "generics" are substantially less expensive.
3. Your doctor may not know the relative merits of a "brand name" versus a "generic" drug in each particular instance but he should be willing to try to find out before he prescribes one or the other.
4. If your doctor finally does prescribe a "generic" drug for you, shop around at different pharmacies for the best price and insist that the pharmacist give you the "generic" product your physician has prescribed.

REFERENCES

1. General Information Report, National Prescription Audit-National Hospital Audit. Ambler, Pennsylvania, Lea, Inc., 1972.
2. Burack, R.: *The New Handbook of Prescription Drugs*. New York, Ballantine Books, 1970.
3. "Cost of Commonly Used Oral Antimicrobials for Adult Infections." *Medical Letter of Drugs and Therapeutics*, volume 13, page 26, 1971.
4. "Oral Antihistamines for Allergic Disorders." Medi-

cal Letter of Drugs and Therapeutics, volume 13, page 104, 1971.
5. Horwitz, R. A., Morgan, J. P., and Fleckenstein, L.: "Savings from Generic Prescriptions." Annals of Internal Medicine, volume 82, page 601, 1975.
6. *Drug Bioequivalence Study Panel Report.* Office of Technology Assessment, Congress of the United States, July 1974, page 1.

2. ANTICIPATING THE COST OF YOUR MEDICAL CARE

One of the frustrating elements of dealing with anyone who provides you with a service is receiving a bill much larger than you expected, especially when you have no way of knowing whether you have been served well. This problem is amplified when the service is health care delivery, because many diseases relentlessly pursue their own course despite any medical intervention. Furthermore, many other diseases go away by themselves and require no significant treatment at all. In these situations, therefore, the physician's service to the patient is really limited to identifying the illness as serious or minor, treatable, untreatable, or not worthy of treatment. No tangible product passes from the physician to the patient in these cases and when the patient receives the doctor's bill he is often puzzled and sometimes angered by its size.

Much of the dissatisfaction which the patient-consumer voices today is directly related to large bills from doctors and hospitals for services which he was not aware of or did not understand. This situation doesn't have to exist. The fact that it does reveals that there is a serious breakdown in communication between the patient and the doctor, or the hospital. Moreover, the patient frequently doesn't understand the extent of his insurance benefits.

There is a simple remedy. Many doctors and hospitals make pamphlets available in waiting rooms or upon request from a receptionist which explain the doctor's or hospital's fees and billing practices. These pamphlets often explain the rationale behind the doctor's basic office visit fee on an hourly scale or some other understandable basis. Other items which should also be listed are the cost of any special procedures performed by the doctor such as proctoscopy; the cost of injections or simple laboratory tests; the cost of house calls (if he makes them); hospital or nursing home visits and the like. If your doctor's office doesn't supply you with this information then it is your responsibility to speak with his staff or with the doctor himself and ask for this information. *Do not be afraid or too embarrassed to ask!* If the fees are reasonable, if the doctor is confident in his own integrity and if he is basically dedicated to serving his patients, he will be neither offended nor angry. In fact, from a business point of view he should be pleased; for if a patient knows roughly what the fees are likely to be and willingly remains in that doctor's practice, the doctor is generally assured that he will have little trouble collecting those fees.

The other area which oftentimes shocks patients is the unexpectedly large size of hospital bills, even for relatively brief periods of hospitalization. Although the patient can occasionally exert some control over the size of the bill he gets from his doctor, there is usually very little he can do to modify the hospital bill. However, you should be able to find out, before you enter the hospital, what its basic daily charges are. You should also inquire about the cost of regularly provided services such as: medications; intravenous fluid solutions; wound dressings; blood transfusions; oxygen tents, tanks and masks; special duty nursing care; operating room, recovery room and intensive care unit services; special diagnostic equipment; electrocardiograms; x-rays; physical and occupational therapy; common laboratory tests, and so on. Many hospitals can also tell you what the average length of stay and average hospital costs are for a variety of common illnesses. This should help to give you a rough idea of how much a particular hospital stay will cost.

If you have any questions after you have gotten the bill you should not hesitate to ask someone in the billing office to explain the reason for any charge that isn't perfectly clear to you. Since many hospitals use a code for each of their charges there may be little or no way for you to understand what any of the charges are for. You are entitled, therefore, to have the entire bill explained to you, line by line, if you so desire. *Don't be afraid to ask for this; you have a right to know what you are paying for.* In summary:

1. You have a right to know what a doctor's or hospital's fee structure is like before you engage their services.

Don't hesitate to ask for this information. Most physicians and hospitals are happy to oblige.
2. The bill you receive from your physician or hospital should be itemized and the nature and price of each item should be clearly listed for your information. If they aren't, you are entitled to a thorough explanation before you pay. Mistakes and duplications do sometimes occur so check the bill carefully.

If you use this approach you will be able to understand, anticipate and budget for your medical expenses. The costs of medical care today are too high to do otherwise.

3. ESSENTIALS OF AN ADEQUATE HEALTH INSURANCE PLAN

As this book goes to print no National Health Insurance program has been signed into law but it appears that approval of one program or another will occur during the next few years. Because of the imminence of this historical decision and because it is well beyond the scope of this book, we will not discuss the commercial health insurance industry. We will only point out what we consider to be the absolutely essential features that any good health insurance plan, private or federal, should provide for the consumer.

1. It should be noncancellable. In other words, the company should be unable to cancel the policy for any reason

other than nonpayment of premiums or, if you participate in a group policy, leaving the group.
2. It should cover you fully in case of catastrophic illness. Most basic health insurance policies have a limit on the number of dollars they will pay for your health care in any given year. Therefore, in addition to a basic plan you should also have a policy which covers you for at least 80 percent of the costs incurred over this limit—due, for example, to major surgery followed by prolonged hospitalization and intensive therapy.
3. It should have a reasonably low deductible clause, e.g., $100 per year.
4. It should be comprehensive and cover you and your family for all legitimate medical and surgical expenses including the full costs of obstetrical care.

We emphasize that these are bare minimum requirements. If you want reliable information about which private insurance carrier in your area provides the most comprehensive coverage, check with the director of the business office at your local hospital.

10

Advice to the Dissatisfied Consumer

THERE IS A GREAT DEAL of consumer dissatisfaction with the medical profession today, some justified and some not. One has only to listen to the radio, watch TV talk shows, read the newspaper, or talk to his neighbor to hear these complaints. They usually have something to do with the physician's fees, his billing policy, his unavailability and his manner. Much less often the complaint concerns the physician's competence. What is surprising is that very little of this dissatisfaction ever reaches the physician directly from his irate patient in his office. What is not surprising in this setting is that if the physician hears about his patient's dissatisfaction at all it is often through his lawyer in a courtroom.

One of the most serious flaws in our society today is the breakdown in meaningful interpersonal communication. Despite great technological advances which have made nearly instantaneous transglobal conversation possible, there has been progressive deterioration in man's ability to be open, candid and caring toward his neighbor. We suspect that the increasing mobility of society and the intrusion of faceless corporations into many consumer service areas have been major forces which prevent people from getting to know each other well. Whatever the cause, the illness is manifest in society at large in the form of increasing divorce rates, a demand for consumer protection services (people asking faceless agencies to protect them from the abuses of other faceless agencies) and rising numbers of medical malpractice suits.

Let us examine the area of malpractice suits more closely, since we believe that their rising incidence is a symptom of a serious breakdown in physician-patient communication due in part to the changing nature of the practice of medicine and the mobility of the average American consumer. This theory is supported by the fact that the cost of malpractice insurance is lowest in New Hampshire, where the population is relatively stable and communities are small enough so that patients are likely to know their physicians reasonably well on many different levels. In contrast, malpractice insurance rates are highest in California, with its notoriously mobile population and sprawling communities.

It is easy to imagine how easily the following common situation contributes to extreme consumer dissatisfaction with malpractice litigation as its natural consequence. John Doe received an unexpectedly high bill from his doctor several years ago. He was quite upset about this but, since his insurance company paid most of the bill and since he was too busy to take the time to discuss the bill with the physician, he paid his share and said nothing. The seed of resentment, however, was planted.

A few years later, now in a different state, he was forced to wait for over two hours in a physician's waiting room while his head was pounding from a severe headache and he was severely nauseated with an intestinal viral infection. When he finally got in to see the busy physician, he was treated somewhat brusquely, told that he had a minor viral illness and dismissed in less than five minutes with instructions to take aspirin, get plenty of rest and drink only clear liquids. Because he felt so sick and because the doctor made it clear that he was pressed for time, Mr. Doe left the office filled with suppressed hostility.

Some time later he read about a disreputable group of doctors who were under indictment for trying to defraud the government of Medicare funds. His feelings of frustration, resentment and hostility which had been building up over the years now seemed to him to be justified and his opinion of all physicians and the medical profession fell to an all-time low.

Then one day his daughter fell down a flight of stairs and cut her face. He took her to the nearest emergency room, where the nurse managed to get the bleeding stopped. Mr. Doe and his daughter had to wait for over an hour for the doctor on call, whom they didn't know, to arrive. The physician sewed up the cut, gave the child a tetanus shot, told Mr. Doe to have the stitches removed in a few days, and departed. Again infuriated by this lack of concern but too embarrassed to speak up, he and his daughter left. The wound didn't heal properly, however, and the child was left with a noticeable scar. Without giving it a second thought, Mr. Doe decided he had been mistreated enough by the medical profession and headed straight to his lawyer's office and began malpractice proceedings.

This example is certainly not meant to deny the fact that medical negligence and incompetence exist and that under some circumstances the patient is justified in initiating a lawsuit. We intend it, rather, to dramatize how feelings of hostility and resentment can build up over the years, slowly reach the boiling point and suddenly explode in the face of a relatively minor incident. In many cases the factor that precipitates the malpractice suit is like the proverbial straw that broke the camel's back. It is the match that finally ignites the years of accumulated resentment.

This situation needn't exist, and there is a great deal that you, the consumer, can do to prevent it from happening to you. First, and most important, you can use the methods outlined in Chapter 1 to evaluate the background, training, competence and office practices of the physician you select. You should be discriminating in this decision because it is the most important decision you will make regarding not only the professional quality of your health care but also the personal manner in which it is dispensed. Second, you should never allow any sort of misunderstanding between you and your physician to pass without making a serious effort to discuss it with him.

Because of their busy schedules most physicians usually are unaware that they or one of their staff have offended a patient. Indeed, in an effort to spend more time with individual patients some physicians are limiting the number of patients they see each day. Others are employing physicians' assistants to improve the efficiency of their practices. A concerned physician will want to know how he has offended you and will usually explain how the situation arose and apologize. Physicians, like most other people, are basically decent individuals. If, however, you are rebuffed when you try to discuss the problem with your physician you shouldn't let your discontent fester within you. Mechanisms already exist within the system which are designed to allow consumers to express their specific grievances, to invesitgate these complaints and to censure the offending physician.

The County or State Medical Societies in your area have Grievance Committees which exist specifically to hear and review complaints against their members. Most practicing physicians belong to these societies. Therefore, if your physician refuses to discuss your complaint personally you have the right to report him to the local medical society. We view this option as more than a right. To our way of thinking, if the reasonable consumer can't discuss a difference of opinion with his physician, it is likely that other patients in that doctor's practice are also dissatisfied. The patient who reports this physician is, therefore, doing himself and others a favor. Furthermore, he will be assisting the medical profession to police itself.

The local medical society has the power to publicly

censure a physician, eject him from membership in the society, or refer the case to the State Board of Medical Examiners. The State Board, in turn, has similar powers and, in addition, can revoke a physician's license to practice. The pressure that this public awareness places on physicians is considerable and, if it is widespread, can result in a greater responsiveness on the part of physicians to their patients' needs. This in turn will improve the quality of medical care, decrease the number of malpractice suits and ultimately reduce the cost of a visit to your doctor as his malpractice insurance rate falls.

In summary:

1. Consumer dissatisfaction with medical care today is primarily due to inadequate communication between patient and physician.
2. If communication is improved, the patient and the physician will be better able to understand and appreciate the reasons behind the needs and demands they make on each other and dissatisfaction will diminish to their mutual benefit.
3. If you have a significant grievance with your physician you should make every effort to discuss the matter with him.
4. If a physician is unresponsive to these requests or if he fails to correct the situation you owe it to yourself, your neighbor and the medical profession to report him to the Grievance Committee of your County or State Medical Society. By so doing you are performing the vital function of helping the medical profession police itself.
5. If these practices become widespread, physicians in gen-

eral will be more responsive to the patient's needs, dissatisfaction will diminish, malpractice suits will decrease, malpractice insurance premiums will fall and physicians' fees should fall accordingly.

Although the practice of medicine will never return to the days of the old-fashioned country physician, the doctor-patient relationship can still be warm, pleasant and therapeutic. If both parties take a moment to analyze the forces at work in society that interfere with this relationship, and realize how fragile and yet how important this relationship really is to the patient's health and the physician's reputation, perhaps it can be salvaged. By being bold enough to discuss his complaints directly with his physician the patient automatically declares how important the relationship is to him. If the physician doesn't respond in a way which will preserve the relationship, it should be terminated. If he does, the relationship will have been strengthened.

Appendix

HOME MEDICAL LIBRARY

Each family should have a health library. There are several excellent and authoritative books which define and explain the symptoms and treatment of various diseases. We recommend that you obtain the following books for your home:

1. *The Merck Manual*, 12th edition, Merck and Co., Rahway, NJ, 1972. This is a classic medical text which describes diseases, signs and symptoms, and lists conventional therapeutic regimens.

This book is often used by medical students and physicians in training but is written clearly enough for the layman to understand.

2. *AMA Drug Evaluations* (prepared by the American

Medical Association Department of Drugs), 2nd edition, Publishing Sciences Group, Acton, MA, 1973.

This is a clear and concise description of commonly used drugs, when they should be used, when avoided and side effects. Most of your questions about specific illnesses can be answered if this book and The Merck Manual are used together.

3. *Baby and Child Care,* by Benjamin Spock, M.D., Pocket Books, Inc., New York, NY.

The classic and eminently practical guide to child health and development. An indispensable aid to parents of young children. Will save you many unnecessary visits to the doctor's office.

4. *The Medicine Show: Consumer's Union Practical Guide to Some Every Day Health Problems and Health Products,* by the editors of Consumer's Report, Consumer's Union, Mt. Vernon, NY, 1974.

5. *Your Medicare Handbook,* DHEW Publication No. (SSA) 74-10050, Social Security Administration, Washington, DC.

Describes the extent of coverage and ground rules of the Medicare program.

REFERENCE BOOKS

The following books are available in most large public libraries on a reference basis:

A. Information about Drugs

1. *Handbook of Non-Prescription Drugs*, American Pharmaceutical Association, Washington, DC, 1973.
2. *Physicians' Desk Reference*, Medical Economics, Oradell, NJ, 1975.
3. Goodman, L. S., and Gilman, A.: *The Pharmacologic Basis of Therapeutics*, 4th edition, The Macmillan Co., NY, 1970.

B. Information about your Physician and Hospital

1. *Directory of Medical Specialists*, A. N. Marquis Co., Chicago, IL, 1974–75.

    An excellent list of board certified physicians, their education and training and the requirements for board certification.
2. *U.S. Physician Reference Listing* (14 volumes), Fisher-Stevens, Inc., Clifton, NJ, 1973.
3. *American Hospital Association Guide to the Health Care Field*, American Hospital Association, Chicago, IL, volume published annually.

    A list of hospitals and nursing homes which summarizes the services they offer, accreditation and other important information.

C. Information about Allied Health Personnel

1. *Allied Health Medical Education Directory*, Council on Medical Education, American Medical Association, 1974.

D. Information about Health Insurance

1. *What you Should Know about Health Insurance*, Health Insurance Institute, 1975.

Pocket Health Record

The following outline is designed to provide an attending physician with vital information about your health during an emergency situation, especially if you are unconscious. Study it carefully and have your doctor help you fill it out if necessary. Keep it with you at all times.

NAME: *RACE:*   *SEX:*
ADDRESS:
DATE OF BIRTH: *SOCIAL SECURITY NO.:*
HEIGHT: *WEIGHT:*
EYE COLOR: *HAIR COLOR:*
BLOOD TYPE: *RELIGION:*

HEALTH INSURANCE COMPANY:
POLICY NO.:
MEDICARE NO.:   *MEDICAID NO.:*
NEXT OF KIN
  Name:
  Address:
  Phone:
PERSONAL PHYSICIAN
  Name:
  Address:
  Phone:
LAST TETANUS BOOSTER:
ALLERGIES
Type (e.g. Penicillin, Bee Sting, etc)
Symptoms (e.g. Rash, Wheezing)
DATE OF LAST PREGNANCY:
PROFILE OF MAJOR ILLNESSES

HEART DISEASE

  Type:
  Medications (Include Dose):
  Last Check-up:
  Physician and Phone No.:
  Related Surgery:
  Surgeon and Phone No.:

CANCER

Type:
Medications:
Last Check-up:
Physician and Phone No.:
Related Surgery:
Surgeon and Phone No.:

DIABETES

Age at Onset:
Medications:
   Type of Insulin: *Dose:*   *How Often:*
   Oral Drugs: *Dose:*   *How Often:*
Complications:
  Diabetic Coma (Ketoacidosis)
  Insulin Reaction (Hypoglycemia)
  Gangrene
  Heart Attack
  Stroke
  Blindness
  Kidney Disease
  Physician and Phone No.:

EPILEPSY

Type:
Medications:
Physician and Phone No.:

HIGH BLOOD PRESSURE

LAST CHECK-UP	
BLOOD PRESSURE	
DRUGS & DOSE	
LAST CHECK-UP	
BLOOD PRESSURE	
DRUGS & DOSE	
LAST CHECK-UP	
BLOOD PRESSURE	
DRUGS & DOSE	

Complications:
- *Heart Disease*
- *Stroke*
- *Aneurysm*
- *Kidney Disease*
- *Dizziness*
- *Blurred Vision*
- *Physician and Phone No.:*

STROKE

Type:
- *Hemorrhage*
- *Blood Clot*

Paralysis:
- *Right Arm*
- *Left Arm*
- *Right Leg*
- *Left Leg*
- *Right Side of Face*
- *Left Side of Face*

Speech:

Vision:
Medications:
Physician and Phone No.:

INTESTINAL BLEEDING

		Number
Reason:	Date:	No. Transfusions

Esophageal Varices
Stomach Ulcer
Stomach Cancer
Duodenal Ulcer
Colitis
Colon Cancer
Diverticulosis
Hemorrhoids
Other

Medications:
Physician and Phone No.:
Most Recent Hematocrit:
Date:
Related Surgery:
Surgeon and Phone No.:

KIDNEY DISEASE

Type:
Medications:
Last B.U.N. and Date:
Last Creatinine and Date:
Dialysis?
Transplant?
Physician and Phone No.:

OTHER MAJOR ILLNESSES

Disease   *Medications*

Anemia
Cirrhosis
Emphysema
Bronchitis
Tuberculosis in Past?
Asthma
Pulmonary Embolism
Hyperthyroidism
Hypothyroidism

Tetany
Glaucoma
Bleeding Tendency
Addison's Disease
Myasthenia Gravis
Psychiatric Illness
Attempted Suicide
Spontaneous Pneumothorax
Physician and Phone No.

OTHER GENERAL INFORMATION

List All Previous Surgery, Date, Surgeon and Phone No.:

List All Current Medications and Dose:

List Known Abnormal Laboratory Tests: